Eat Yoga!

Eat Yoga!

The Only Guidebook for Life You'll Ever Need

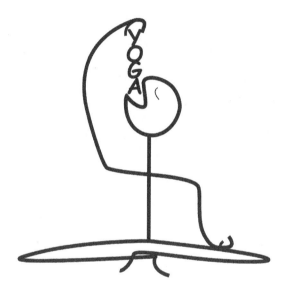

by

DH Parsons

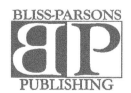

BLISS-PARSONS
PUBLISHING

EAT YOGA!
The Only Guidebook for Life You'll Ever Need

Disclaimer:

The author of this book does not, either directly or indirectly, dispense medical advice, nor does he prescribe the use of any technique or form of treatment for physical or medical problems without the advice of a physician. The intent of the author is to provide support and encouragement for your personal, physical, and spiritual health and well-being. Should you choose to apply any of the information in this book to yourself, as is your right, you do so at your own discretion. The author and publisher assume no responsibility for your actions.

ISBN: 978-0-9963176-7-2

Library of Congrees Control Number: 2017919054

This book is dedicated to all the students and friends who have graced my classes over the years, and to all those who will adopt the lifestyle outlined on these pages and move forward in happiness and in health.

Also by DH Parsons:

The Diary of Mary Bliss Parsons
Volume 1: The Strong Witch Society
Volume 2: The Lost Revelation
Volume 3: Beyond Infinite Healing
published by All Things That Matter Press

The Muse: Coming of Age in 1968
published by Bliss-Parsons Publishing

About the Author

DH Parsons, author, artist, internationally known intuitive, and educator, has been practicing and teaching yoga for over fifty years and is well known throughout the yoga community. This handbook was written in response to numerous requests from students and friends. It is a concise and informative distillation of yogic science, philosophy, and practice, and includes advice and instruction for a life of enhanced physical health and spiritual well-being.

In addition to his extensive background and training in yoga, his credentials include a bachelor's degree in art, a master's degree in education, doctoral degrees in comparative religion and metaphysics, and service as a public and private school teacher (art, journalism, English, and history), high school dean of students, and middle school administrator.

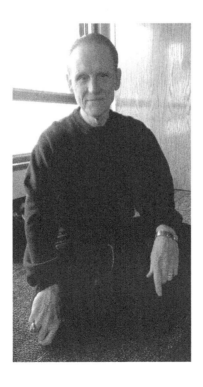

Contents

Preface
Why Did I Get Into Yoga In the First Place?

I was born with bronchial asthma, so throughout my youth I could do none of the things the other kids did—run rough and tumble in country fields, play sports, join organizations with activities centered around the raising of and caring for animals. My participation in any of those activities resulted in sucking up dust, pollen, and animal dander into my lungs, and would end with a trip to the hospital.

It seemed like everything I did brought on an asthma attack—and this was long before the convenient rescue inhalers were invented. When I was nine years old, a particularly bad attack evolved into full-blown double pneumonia. I wound up in the hospital in serious condition for nearly two weeks, culminating in a near death experience (the doctor reported that I had been without breath or heartbeat for about a minute), a miraculous recovery, and a train trip to Southern California.

On the bright side, my asthma forced me to take myself in directions most kids would never think of going. Instead of spending time and effort to become a baseball star or a veterinarian, my energies were focused inward. I read voraciously and my imagination took me into worlds I might never have dreamed of had I been like everyone else. I studied Egyptian, Greek, and Celtic mythologies and sought for deeper meanings within those ancient cultures. I read and studied the Bible until I could quote scripture with the best of them at the age of fourteen. I dove into other religions and philosophies as well, including those of Japan, China, and India. It was during my study of Indian history and culture that I became interested in the art and science of yoga.

I don't remember the title of the first book about yoga that came into my possession. I do remember that it had lots of pictures of a plump Indian man placing himself into postures that were almost impossible for my young head to understand, let alone for my body to imitate. What impressed me most in that book was finding out that those postures were used not only to make the body healthier, but also to make the mind more alert. I learned, too, that true yoga is an exercise demanding not so much physical exertion, but more mental discipline, and that when practiced, is beneficial to one's entire being—physical, mental, and spiritual. What's more, the book promised that if the practitioner applied him or herself diligently to the mental exercise, then the physical health benefits would naturally be stimulated in the body with little physical exertion at all.

Well, being a weak skinny kid with asthma, that all sounded pretty good to me! So I decided I would investigate this yoga thing in earnest. I figured the best way to approach my new interest was to try to find more books on yoga and study them from cover to cover.

This part of my life took place in the early to mid 1960s, when yoga was just beginning to emerge from its early counterculture obscurity into the awareness of the American general public. The 60s also saw the beginning of the expansion of health food stores, vegetarianism, and fitness centers into the mainstream of culture. Yoga was one of those new, "hip, in, and groovy" things that would eventually morph into the billion-dollar fitness industry we have today.

I was able to find a few books in the bookstore in those early years that proved to be of more practical use than my first one. I brought them home, opened them up, and got lost in them; the rest is history.

By the time I entered high school, I had lost some of the fragility of my earlier childhood. I still spent much of my time after school and on weekends in solitary and mostly sedentary pursuits, such as studying, reading, writing, and getting lost in the travels of my mind. I didn't watch much TV—there wasn't much to watch back then—but I occasionally caught a football game. I wasn't really attracted to the sport, but I was fascinated by and envious of any human who was able to participate in such a rough and tumble sport without having his lungs shut down.

After watching one of those games I decided I'd try out for the freshman football team. Lots of other kids, some of them fairly scrawny, were going out for it too, so it seemed like the thing to do.

Even though I wasn't really into sports I did think it would be pretty cool to be one of the jocks. I don't think it had much to do with wanting to be a big muscle-bound stud, or to look like Joe Namath and get all the girls; I think it had more to do with the uniform, and especially those neat little shoes with cleats the football players all wore. I figured that if I just owned a pair of those shoes, and if I could carry them around school slung over my shoulder like the jocks did, I'd be a jock too!

So, the first thing I did, even before I attended a single day of football practice, was order a pair of those neato football cleats, COD (cash on delivery). I remember how disappointed I was when they told me it would take three weeks to get the shoes in the mail. That was okay though, because the coach told us we would be practicing in tennis shoes for a while and we wouldn't need them right away.

The day after I ordered my cleats, football practice began — and it just about killed me. There I was, a short, over-weight and getting fatter little kid, and I was expected to share the practice field with eighty or ninety guys all named Bubba, or Jake. And they were huge! Of course, they were not all freshman; some were already on the jv team or the varsity team, but we all used the same fields for our practice.

I did a lot of yoga breathing that day in anticipation of what might occur out on the field. Asthma was the least of my concerns; I was about to come into hard contact with those monsters, some of whom were six feet tall and weighed 200 pounds or more. Several of them had only one eyebrow that stretched shaggily from the top of one ear to the other, and they all seemed to communicate in sentences of one or two syllable sentences like, "Unnngh," and, "Ommmph Pah Ugh."

For three days I hacked and wheezed and pounded my body against large things like potato sacks filled with sawdust or straw. I tackled odd-looking leather objects. I rammed myself into tackle horses, and I slipped and fell and tumbled and had my head knocked around and my arms nearly twisted off all in the name of glory.

It was total insanity.

Finally, on the afternoon of the third day of practice I was tackled hard—really hard—driven to my knees by a 200-pound forehead with an eyebrow the size of St. Louis. Both of my knees were hurt badly; one had to be put into a cast. My football career was over. Three days. Three days of torture, agony, pain, and nonglory. No one called me a jock, and not one girl even looked at me. The day I crawled off that practice field I swore I'd never go out for another sport again.

On my way home from the hospital with my knee in the new cast, I remember thinking to myself over and over and over:

I love yoga. I love yoga. I love yoga.

The football cleats came in the mail three weeks later.

1
Yoga: More Than Just Postures

This is a handbook of yoga for the enhancement of your health and wellbeing. In addition to a sequence of yoga postures, *EAT YOGA!* contains a little bit of history and philosophy. It also contains a lot of information about nutrition and easy to find and prepare foods, a logical and practical diet. You will also find here a simple, life-changing breathing technique. This book is about you and your physical health, and how to make it better without buying any expensive products or trying to fit into one of the faddish yoga classes so popular these days.

The yoga described here is not "power yoga," "hot yoga," or any other modern form of yoga that forces the body into difficult, unnatural and even dangerous contortions while producing lots of sweat. What is presented is a sequence of gentle, classical Hatha yoga postures, with additional movements described to allow the fluid transition from one posture to the next. The result is a graceful routine that is easily performed daily by anyone, regardless of age or physical ability, at any time to suit your own busy schedule.

There are many misconceptions about the practice of yoga. Much of what passes for yoga today is not really yoga, but rather a mixture of calisthenics, difficult postures, aerobics, and sometimes, even gymnastics. Real yoga is an age-old system of physical techniques to be practiced supplementary to a broader program for the improvement of body and mind. Hatha yoga, or simply yoga, as this form has come to be known in the 20th century, is not a religion or a philosophy. It is, however, more than just movement through a series of physical poses. Yoga is a satisfying lifestyle that can bring not only a sense of satisfaction and achievement, but can also bring you to better health in a relatively short period of time.

While Yoga does have links to Hindu tradition—after all, it did originate in India—it is NOT Hinduism. The word *yoga* is from the Sanskrit language, and means *yoke* or *union*. The concept is simple but vital, and transcends fads, philosophies, political boundaries, traditions, and religion. It is universal.

This book also contains dietary and health suggestions, and a little of the history and science of yoga—all of which will help you maximize your own personal practice of yoga, enhancing its benefits along the way. Doing the postures once or twice a week is a good thing, but by understanding some of the history and science behind the postures, you can visualize the physiological effects they are having on you as you do them. If you are anxious to get started with the physical practice of yoga as described in Chapter 7, you may, but I strongly recommend that you read the entire book once before you actually begin your practice. Consider the exercise of learning the background and science of yoga to be a mental discipline that will set the stage for your own growth and renewal as you embark on the *EAT YOGA!* lifestyle.

To Be, or Not To Be: Further arguments in favor of pursuing a yogic lifestyle.

When you ask the question, "What does it mean, *to be*," you get a variety of responses:

"To get up, go to work, come home, go to bed, get up, and go to work again. That's what it means *to be* me."

"*To be* is to be born and to live; and when you die you aren't any more."

"I didn't have a choice! Nobody asked me if I wanted *to be* or not!"

"To have all the fun you can have before you die."

"I love sports. I don't want *to b*e if I can't watch football!"

And my favorite, "What do you mean, *What does it mean?*"

The reason for your existence—for your being or not being—is inherent within you from your birth. It comes at the very moment of your conception, along with the package you call *self*. You just don't recognize it. You have too much on your mind. Society has burdened you with a hefty load of mental, physical and emotional garbage, and every day it seems like a struggle just to stay on top of it. Who has time to think about anything deeper than, "Where are my car keys? I'll be late for work," or, "I hope the computers aren't down again today," or, "I wonder if So-and-So in *Name-Your-Favorite-Series* will die in the next episode."

We live in a fast-paced world that seems to be centered around three elements that have become associated with success in our society: greed, ego, and entertainment. You don't have to dig very deep to find they are some of the strongest drivers of our culture. People in America would rather go to a football game than attend a church or a synagogue. They would rather read all the sordid details about the lives of their favorite entertainers than read one page of the Bible, the Torah, the Bhagavad Gita, *Walden's Pond*, or even one of my books (which aren't all about yoga). They would rather claw their way to the top of the social and workplace ladders, destroying friendships and hurting other people along the way, than make the most of the gifts they have been given while personally giving a hand up to others. Uncontrolled egos would rather punish than praise someone else.

Earlier in my life when I was a school administrator, many of my fellow administrators seemed to take great pleasure in calling their teachers onto the carpet any time there was the slightest slip up. On the other hand, when a teacher did something truly wonderful, the administrators rarely acknowledged the contribution, and often took credit for it themselves. I asked one of my colleagues why he behaved this way; his answer was, "Because I can. I have the power."

The self-centered existence that is so characteristic of modern culture is the product of the willful, collective thought of humanity. The force of it has grown beyond a nebulous malaise to become a destructive energy disconnecting humankind from the essence of life, and threatening to consume its future. Application of the principles and practices set forth in this book can slow or even reverse this destructive path. In order to learn how that can be accomplished, we first need to examine how we got here.

Many of us living in this modern society tend to feel superior to prehistoric man. Our advanced brains have developed technologies that easily take care of our basic needs. Our food is gathered together into central locations, neatly presented to us in clean, convenient packages, and requires little or no preparation prior to consumption. We live in houses that keep us dry and comfortable regardless of the conditions outside, and supply us with clean hot or cold water at a touch. Food, clothing, and entertainment can all be acquired easily and quickly by simply hopping in the car and driving to the grocery store, shopping mall, theater, or sports arena. The type of work we do to earn the money we need to pay for all this is far removed from basic physical survival, and the void of our spare time is often filled with mindless activity that keeps us from contemplating our true nature and our place and purpose in this creation.

On the other hand, all prehistoric man had to do was try to stay alive. After all, he didn't own a computer, watch the Super Bowl, drink beer, text, go to Hot Yoga classes, or hold an administrative position. All he had to do was survive. Yet, it was prehistoric man who asked the first questions such as:

"Why am I here?"

"Is there a God?"

"What is the meaning of life?"

He questioned because he had time to question. When not engaged in the activities necessary for survival—finding food and shelter, warding off predators, et cetera—his mind was free to contemplate his place among the details of the world with which he was intimately familiar. His mind didn't have to compete with all the things modern man believes he must have in order to make him happy. Had the prehistoric man owned the latest computer, perhaps these thoughts would never have occurred in his mind, either. All he would have had to do was hook up to the internet and download information about an infinite number of topics. He could have Googled all day and become just as confused about the meaning of life as most people are today.

Modern man doesn't know what it means *to be*, because he no longer feels his being. His being has been replaced by computers, basketball games, lawsuits, politically correct agendas, recreational drugs, computer games, Hollywood, insipid music, violent movies —the list goes on. Materialism and addictions to ego and entertainment have become his latest religion, and these manifestations of self-centered existence have even invaded modern churches, as well as many of the faddish variations of yoga being offered these days. Human beings are possessed by their possessions and their own self-idolatry. Celebrities have become the human gods, and humans worship their gods every time they score a goal, produce a blockbuster movie, or record their latest adolescent musical performance.

BUT, once in a while a different kind of person emerges from the sea of superficiality. This is a person who feels the compulsion to revive the old questions: "Who am I?" "Who is God?" "What is this all about?" Unfortunately, that person is often labeled a religious fanatic, a cultist, a kook, or a heretic. They are referred to as pagan, naive, simple-minded, or even ignorant.

Some well-known representatives of this class come to mind: Jesus Christ, Galileo, Paramhansa Yogananda, Jonathan Edwards, St. Francis of Assisi, Mahatma Gandhi, Billy Graham, St. Teresa d'Avila, Thomas Merton, Pope John Paul II, Robert Honaker, St. Therese of Lisieux, and many others. All of these naive, simple-minded, and free-thinking folk had a pretty hard time of it at the hands of their critics, simply because they asked those same crazy questions. More importantly, they embodied the kind of yoga that I not only promote and teach in this book and in my yoga classes, but is the same yoga that is the key to being *fully alive*.

So why are humans still asking those crazy, meaning-of-life questions? Is it because they have never been answered? Or is it because the answers are *not* somewhere Out There?

The answers are to be found within your soul and in your spirit — the energies that hold your true identity. You need only to awaken to or become aware of the answers that were given freely by God in the beginning when humans were first placed on this world. But this process of awakening requires the removal of that load of garbage the world has saddled you with.

Religion and History and Yoga, OH MY!

For many people, a spiritual life is all about adopting some austere, self-effacing discipline for the purpose of seeking God—somewhere "out there"—and asking Him to please come down and be with them every Sunday morning for an hour or so while, motivated by fear and superstition, they serve out their time observing the obligatory rituals.

On the contrary, spirituality is the realization that God does not have to be sought after at all, but that He has been with you forever. It is the process of the renewal of your recognition that God is not "out there," but that He is as close as the air you breathe, and that He will share His very Spirit with your own if you only ask. No one has to seek God.

God did not plant humans on this tiny world on the edge of a galaxy in the middle of the nowhere that is deep space, and then speed off into oblivion to leave them on their own. God never left humanity. He could NOT leave because He had chosen to be with humanity for eternity. Even Jesus said, "My Father and I are one." He then went on to say that humans must become a part of that oneness with God, by way of the initial choice to return to it. But first you must understand what it means to be at one with God.

Enter yoga. The ultimate goal of a yogic lifestyle is not merely to achieve glowing physical health—although that is part of it. The ultimate goal is union, or communion with God, and that is what the word *yoga* actually implies. As I said previously, *yoga* literally means *yoke*—as in that big heavy wooden yoke that inseparably binds two oxen together. The word, *yoga* implies an inseparable union with God, in that a person has become yoked together with God in his or her personal life. He or she cannot be separated from God because of their practice of yoga, which constantly insures the connection.

Please note that this is not the same as the idea promoted by many of the modern New Age philosophies. The idea that you literally become God, or that everyone is divine and living on an equal status with God is just one example of a modern reinterpretation of an age-old spiritual truth. God is absolute and unchanging. Unity with God must be consciously chosen and actively pursued. When Jesus spoke of oneness with God, He was speaking of being one in terms of thought, word and deed. A person who is one with God is not a little god in and of himself; he is one in the Spirit of the Will of God — meaning that he not only believes in God as his Creator, but that he also strives to do the Will of God in his own life. That is what yoga is and does. Yoga is a matter of close communion with God — a close relationship with God throughout one's life. I have never met a TRUE yogi who professes to be a god, or to be on the same level as the Creator God, as many of the New Age believers seem to think of themselves. I have always thought that kind of self-image was more than just a little bit presumptuous on the part of many New Agers, and actually contrary to some of their own New Age teachings about controlling one's ego. It is also a highly glorified state of being that is simply not possible to achieve as a human. Regardless of what some may teach or preach, humans are limited in their powers and abilities. If you don't believe me just try creating something out of nothing. You can think as positively as you are able; you can recite all the positive affirmations you want, but you just can't turn a boulder into a Dodge Neon.

Another point that needs clarification is the misconception held by some people that yoga is a fundamental and inseparable part of Hinduism, the great religion of India. Although yoga has been adopted into Hinduism as an integral part of some of its practices, it actually predates the religion of Hinduism by centuries.

Yoga finds its earliest origin in mankind's desire to gain insight into the basic nature of all living things. Yoga is a science, a way of living, and an art form that can be combined with any religion, or spiritual path you may now be following. It doesn't matter if you are a Catholic, Jewish, Southern Baptist, Hindu, Taoist or Zen Buddhist; the principles of yoga can be an enhancement, not a detriment, to your personal faith, beliefs, and self-renewal.

In the yogic lifestyle as described in this book, unity with the Will of God is the highest state a practitioner of yoga can reach. It is the interaction of the soul of the yogin with the Spirit of God, Who, through the teachings of nearly every religion on this world, has given His own promise that He will reside within the temple that the human form is meant to become for Him. Even though the ability to commune with God is inherent in everyone, that ability is often not realized or fully developed, primarily because most of us don't take the time to do it.

Before proceeding further, I must draw the distinction between your *soul* and your *spirit*. Your *spirit* is your eternal being—the essence of you that exists throughout eternity. Your *soul* is who you think you are while you are residing inside your physical body. Your spirit is comprised of pure sentient energy, and it lives forever. Your soul is your conscious mind combined with your personality. When your body dies, your spirit will move on to your eternal life and only a residual piece of your soul in the form of memories will accompany your spirit into your eternal life. So it is not your spirit that needs to interact with the Spirit of God, it is your soul that needs that interaction while it is living in the here and now on planet Earth. It is your soul and your mind that need to receive and interact with the Spirit of God in order to help you muddle through the trials of physical life. The point is that when you commune with God, you are not becoming God yourself, you are simply seeking to yoke your conscious soul-mind to Him so that He can help direct you in all that you do here on Earth.

Paramhansa Yogananda, a great spiritual leader of the yoga tradition, once said:

> *Develop the love of God so that I see in your eyes that you are drunk with God and not asking, "When will I have God?"*
> From a lecture on Divine Love

If you find yourself asking, "When will I have God?" then you are far from communion with God. The true yogin would already know in his or her mind and heart that God listens at all times, and that God is also a part of everything the yogin does, day or night. God is with the yogin while sleeping, eating, smiling, frowning, even while staring up at the night sky and asking, *What, really, is out there?*

A truly spiritually minded person is not searching for the Presence of God. He does not wonder where God resides, because he knows with all his heart that he cannot shake God, no matter how hard he tries. God will always be right there with him as he travels his path to the end.

Humans spend far too much time seeking the God who is already there with them, rather than carrying out the responsibilities God has given to them. They use their "seeking of God" as an excuse for shirking their spiritual duty, usually because their worldly activities are far too excessive.

Health and happiness are not just around the corner, they are with you right here and now. Contentment and peace are not just things to be hoped for, they are realities that can be tapped into today. Enlightenment is not just for gurus and saints, it is for you and for everyone else, but a certain amount of effort is needed to reach the level where you know that is true for you. The old saying, "God helps those who help themselves," is a time-tested truth. If you are willing to show God that you are serious about a true relationship, God will be immediately receptive to that, whether or not you belong to any specific church or religion. If you are content with remaining the way you are, then so be it. But you will never find total communion with God without a serious commitment to understand the truth behind finding God—that is, that He requires no seeking. Yoga will open up your heart and soul to that conclusion.

EAT YOGA! is meant to be a basic handbook on all things yogic. It is a simple how-to manual to give yoga students of all levels of skill and all religious faiths and spiritual persuasions a jump-start into a new life. It comes as a result of being hounded over a period of years by my own yoga students, who seem to believe that I might have the ability to produce a simplified, yet comprehensive and serious treatise on how to walk the walk of a true yogin.

I have been asked many times over the years, "What if I belong to a religion? Can I go to a temple, church, or synagogue and still do yoga?" Of course you can, as do many of the students in my classes. A person carries their belief with them wherever they go—doing healthy yoga exercises is not going to change that. Go to your own place of worship and take part in your own religion, whatever that may be, but take what you've found here in *EAT YOGA!* and share it with your Church friends. It just might change their lives for the better."

A Note About Nomenclature

Throughout this book I will be using the Sanskrit terms for yoga practitioners. A practitioner of yoga is designated generically in Sanskrit as a *yogin*, with *yogi* being the masculine form and *yogini* the feminine. For years I just called everyone a yogi because I didn't know these designations. Personally, I think the term *yogini* sounds more Italian than Indian — like something you'd get at an Italian restaurant with a side of garlic bread. Oh well. Frankly, I don't think it matters much what you call a practitioner of yoga, as long as that person is sincere and not just putting on a show.

> *A true yogi feels the throb of his heart in all hearts; his mind in all minds; his presence in all motion. I will be a true yogi.*
> Paramhansa Yogananda, *Metaphysical Meditations*

2

Atma Jayam^{SM} Yoga Renewal
Self-Victory

*"... you seem to have forgotten your true nature, you have
slipped into a kind of sleep."*
Sri Swami Satchidananda, *The Living Gita.*

Humans have slipped into a kind of sleep; they do not take
the time to pay attention to their inner spirits. As a result, most
people have lost their basic understanding of themselves as spirit
beings. A major effect of the practice of yoga is that of awakening
to one's own true nature. This awakening has nothing to do with
religion and is easily achieved.

The key to awakening lies in the ability to reconnect the body
and mind with the spirit self, while maintaining the awareness
that one's true self is not the body or the mind. If you are able to
plug the principles of Yoga into your daily world — make it your
lifestyle, which is what this book is all about — you will learn to
distinguish between the ordinary mental and physiological functions of your material self from your true spiritual nature. When
you do that, you will have achieved atma jayam — self-victory. As
an Atma Jayam Yogin there is nothing you cannot do. Remember
the old *Kung Fu* TV series? Remember how Kwai Chang Caine,
a.k.a. Grasshopper, moved about from town to town while simply
being an observer of all things? He watched, he listened, he learned,
and he used his knowledge to better the world around him. This
is the way of the yogin. This is the way of a *jivanmukta*, one who
has acquired and assimilated self-knowledge. The jivanmukta is the
personification of the art and science of yoga. He or she *is* yoga.
As Krishna states in chapter two of the Bhagavad Gita, he or she
has become "perfection in action."

Remember also that you are only what you perceive yourself
to be in your own mind. The more you train your mind, the more
you can see yourself in any role you wish. You can fulfill your vision

of yourself in a relatively short time if you really put your mind to it. The practice of yoga will help you recognize what part of you will develop as a spiritual and life-affirming being and, conversely, what part of your mind will keep you from achieving your potential.

This is not just positive affirmation or the "power of positive thinking." Positive affirmation is nothing more than wishful thinking unless action is brought into the picture. People who succeed in business, or politics, or even the arts, don't get there by sitting around the house all day speaking positive affirmations. They have a vision. Yes, they *see* themselves as a future president, or a famous artist, or whatever, and there isn't a day that goes by in which they don't tell themselves, "I *will* be successful! There is *nothing* that can stop me!"

More importantly, successful people give it everything they've got. They put their positive thoughts into physical action; that's what Krishna meant by "perfection in action." That's what the Apostle James meant when he wrote, "Faith without works is a dead faith." (James 2:26) You have to put a little work into it.

So let us ask this question: If it works for the businessman and the artist, can it not work even more effectively for those who have even higher goals? The sky is not the limit for the yogin. The feeling that comes with material or physical success in life cannot compare to the feeling one gets when one first becomes aware of the Presence of God during a time of quiet contemplation. Money cannot buy this experience. No amount of power or status can tempt a true yogin to leave the path once this incredible connection has been made. Once the link has been made, the soul of the seeker experiences a renewal of life, or a return to the truth of what Life really is. Like water flowing to the sea, it begins as a single drop of water, but soon grows to becomes a mighty river. The river, that is, the seeker's soul, is drawn as if by gravity to God, the Ocean, in communion, communication, and commitment.

Yoga is about renewal. To renew something means to restore it to its original intention or design. It does not mean to simply get a second wind, update something, or mentally attempt to start over. The true meaning of the word implies that what one had in the beginning was the exact and perfect thing that one was supposed to have, and that somewhere along the way it got all fouled up and now it needs to be renewed. It needs to be returned to its original, perfect, and pure state.

In order to experience your own personal renewal you must first admit to yourself that you *need* to be renewed. Many people in this world refuse to admit that there is anything wrong in their lives. Before long, the lack of a deeper spiritual experience—the understanding of one's self as a spirit connected to all life and to the Creator—manifests as negativity, loss of purpose, and dissatisfaction. Because there is no foundation of spiritual understanding, there is a breakdown between personal relationships, resulting in the familial, societal, and national discord that is spreading throughout our world.

Sooner or later, every person needs to experience a complete renewal, be it physical, spiritual, or a combination of both, and yoga provides a pathway for that.

A Brief History of Yoga

Many years ago, around 200 BC, the great Hindu mystic, Patanjali, devised a system of metaphysical philosophies and physical exercises for the purpose of bringing a human being to a higher awareness of one's own self, and of one's relationship to the Creator. He called this system, Ashtanga Yoga. "Ashtanga" means "eight-limbed," or "eight-branched," like the limbs or branches on a tree. I like to think of these as the rungs of ladder; as one climbs up the ladder, one comes closer to spiritual awareness or attunement and a life of quality, truth and meaning.

Patanjali believed that if a person were to practice the principles of each of these branches or rungs, that person would be able not only to live a truly wonderful physical lifestyle, but also to attain spiritual enlightenment as a result of the discipline exercised in the effort. Keep in mind that Patanjali was addressing the science of yoga, not religion. The word *spiritual* tends to be over used these days and usually refers to religion, but you don't have to be religious to be spiritual. You can attain spiritual enlightenment or awakening without ever setting foot in a church or a temple.

The Eight Limbs, or Rungs, of the Yoga Ladder

1. **Yama**: the restrictions, "don'ts," or "thou shalt not's," of Yoga.
2. **Niyama**: the practices, "do's," or "thou shallt's," of Yoga.
   - The principles of the Yamas and Niyamas are discussed in greater detail in **Chapter 4**, as I believe them to be important to the success or failure of leading a serious Yoga lifestyle.
3. **Asana**: the physical postures one might encounter in a Hatha Yoga class (**Chapter 7**).
4. **Pranayama**: breathing and energy control.
   - A guide for deep breathing is included near the end of **Chapter 6**.
5. **Pratyahara**: control of the senses through the interiorizing of the mind, a practice which aids the overcoming of attachment to desires.
6. **Dharana**: total concentration; centering of the mind; eliminating disturbances and random thoughts in preparation for meditation or prayer.
7. **Dhyana**: the state of true, pure meditation or prayer; a state of near-breathlessness where one is in deep communion with the Creator.
   - Practices promoting Pratyahar, Dharana, and Dhyana are covered in **Chapter 6**.
8. **Samadhi**: the ultimate physical goal. It is a state achieved when one finally "touches" one's own soul to the outermost border of the "Glow" of the Spirit of God in the deepest form of communion a physical human being can attain with God.

If these steps are practiced faithfully, all true yogins will eventually climb at least the first seven rungs over their time on the yoga path. The last rung is more difficult to attain, but it is possible if the heart is pure and the desire is strong. Each step upward brings increasing rewards in the form of physical health and spiritual contentment. Each level of achievement puts you far beyond where you were when you started your journey in life.

In addition to these eight rungs of yoga, there are several sets of disciplines, all of which comprise the main science of yoga known as "Raja yoga," or "Royal yoga", encompassing everything that has to do with the yogic lifestyle. When one makes the commitment to the first seven rungs of the ladder, one's life will naturally be carried into this kind of deeper understanding of Raja yoga. Keep in mind that the purpose of this chapter is to provide you with some background information, not to give you a list of qualifications to check off as if you were earning a merit badge.

The Five Paths of Yoga

Each of the five paths of yoga provide the yogin with a way to tailor their practice to their individual needs, abilities, and personalities. Each one presents a different focus or discipline as a guide to defining and achieving one's physical and spiritual goals. These brief descriptions are intended to give you a better understanding of the totality of yoga as you take the first steps on a path of improved physical and spiritual health and wellbeing, not to turn you into a monk.

As you progress along the path of yoga you will probably want to learn more about the five forms for yourself, and maybe even adopt one or more of them as your own guiding discipline.

1. Bhakti Yoga: the practice of total devotion to God.

Some yogins spend an entire lifetime on this discipline alone, sacrificing even the postures and the breathing techniques along the way. Bhakti yoga cultivates the ability to see the Presence of God in all living things, recognizing the Divinity of Creator over the created, and resulting in a total, complete, sacrificial love of God. This kind of yoga goes above and beyond mere ritual and, again, has nothing to do with Hinduism or any other religion. There are devoted Christians who practice this discipline, as demonstrated by the lives of the lives of St. Francis of Assisi and Billy Graham, for example.

2. Gyana or Jnana Yoga: the yoga of wisdom.

Wisdom in this sense means to be able to distinguish truth in the midst of non-truth. To be able to discern maya (illusion) from reality is Jnana yoga. To learn to recognize and to implement in your life true happiness rather than the false happiness based on cultural norms and societal acceptance is Jnana yoga.

3. Hatha Yoga: the physical practice of the asanas, pranayama, and concentration.

I have combined elements of hatha yoga with elements of kriya yoga to form the basis of Atma Jayam^SM Yoga, which I developed and have been teaching for many years in my classes and workshops, and the principles of which comprise the core of this book.

4. Karma Yoga: the yoga of physical work and discipline.

This discipline teaches the yogin the importance of doing things not just for self, but also for the Creator and all of creation. Sweeping floors, washing the dishes, going to work, paying your bills, all are a part of Karma Yoga. Karma Yoga sees the influence of God in all things, even the most mundane activities of life.

5. Kriya Yoga: the yoga of meditation, contemplation and prayer.

You are a kriya yogin if you have implemented these three practices into your life and do them faithfully on a daily basis. Each of these will add to your physical, mental, and spiritual wellbeing.

Raja Yoga: the blending together of all of the other five Forms of Yoga.

The word *raja* means *royal*. Raja yoga is all of the five forms working together in harmony. A raja yogin is one who is committed to all five yoga disciplines, internalizing the principles of each and applying them to all aspects of his or her daily life. Many strive for this level of yoga commitment, but few attain it. It is best to pick one of the five forms and focus on that one alone. Simplicity usually leads to perfection and success sooner than biting off too much and attempting to make it all work.

3

What Do You Mean, "Eat Yoga"?

"In the beginning was the Word, and the Word was with God, and the Word was God."
John 1:1

People of all faiths will recognize these words as they comprise one of the most familiar verses in the Bible. It has been quoted, misquoted, paraphrased, and manipulated as the basis for countless Sunday morning sermons, discourses and lectures. It has been read and recited for hundreds of years. It is such a short and simple statement, but I can't imagine that the apostle John had any idea how it would be so misused by pastors and pagans alike. When it comes right down to it, from guru to saint, and from prophet to professor, even after all the articulation, conjecture, and hypothesizing, the fact remains that nobody knows what this verse really means. We humans today can only offer a guess, and then go from there.

I won't add to those previous postulations of the true meaning of John's words. Instead, I'm going to assume that it is not necessary to paraphrase, read into, add to, or take away from the literal implication of the verse. I'm going to assume that it means exactly what it says and take it literally.

So, what does this have to do with yoga? Bear with me while I clarify.

Chapter One of the Book of Genesis tells us that, *"In the beginning God created the heaven and the Earth,"* and that He did it all by *speaking* them into existence. In short, as the Words issued forth from God's Mouth, things happened. Things appeared. Things that were never there before were, all of a sudden, there. All from the act of being spoken into being by the Words of God.

This is not such a difficult concept for us to understand if we consider the consequences of our own words. We all know the power that gossip has to illicit intense emotion, to initiate verbal reaction, or retaliatory action—in short, to create moods and movements that weren't there before. The destructive activity of gossiping literally speaks these negative consequences into existence, so to speak. On the other hand, we all know how words of love can motivate dramatic changes in lifestyles and behavior.

This brings to mind the well-known and simple experiment of observing the growth of the "love/hate sunflowers": Two sunflower seeds are planted in identical physical conditions. Containers, soil, and nutrients are matched; sunlight and water are carefully monitored and administered equally. The only difference is that they are each subjected to emotional energies of opposite extremes. One seed is lavished with love, kind expressions, and gentle touches. The plant grows strong, straight, and beautiful. The other seed is cursed, told it is ugly and worthless; it grows weakly and dies quickly.

Consider these observations in light of your own self-regard and in your interactions with others, especially children and other dependent creatures in your care. It may shock you. Whatever disharmonies are present in your personal life and in your family stem largely from the way you think and what comes from your lips.

The truth is that words have consequences; forgetting that truth has made you, your family, and those around you victims by stopping the flow of true love that comes through us from God.

Words have power. Words — spoken, written, or implied — are the physical manifestation of the fundamental nature or essence that comprise them, and that essence is energy. It is a scientific fact that everything in the universe is made of energy; from people to plants, from skyscrapers to automobiles, from the fire you use to cook your food, to the ice you use to preserve it. Everything, without exception, is made from, held together, and powered by energy in one form or another.

The energy at the core of human words is the same energy on a tiny scale that God used to speak life into existence on planet Earth. That energy is more than just a word, it is an actual physical substance. It is that mysterious, supernatural, energetic substance and the process that results from the releasing of it that goes into making all of creation. Once again, do not confuse this with positive affirmations. This is a matter of physics, not of wishing and hoping.

Yes, this is a rather lengthy lead into a discussion on the yogic way of life, and many of you are probably saying to yourselves, "Just get to the point!" Believe me, this little bit of groundwork will help you understand just how it is that yoga works. And, don't worry, this is the most esoteric chapter in the book. Don't worry if you are not scientifically inclined and do not fully understand what follows. Rest assured that it is not necessary that you do so in order to live a yogic lifestyle, or to continue on with this book. I'm just throwing it in because there might be some who are curious about some of the science behind the art.

Familiarize yourself with the following words and their definitions while keeping in mind that this is a book about yoga.

- **Atom**: the smallest particle of a chemical element that can exist alone or in combination with other elements.
- **Molecule**: a group of atoms that are fused together into the smallest foundational component of a chemical compound that is able to participate in a chemical reaction.
- **Nucleus**:
  In **physics**, it is the central core of an atom.
  In **biology**, it is the dense body within a cell that contains the genetic material.
- **Proton**: the positively charged subatomic particle present in all atomic nuclei.
- **Electron**: the negatively charged subatomic particle orbiting the nucleus of an atom. Electrons determine the electrical, thermal, optical and magnetic properties of substances, and the flow of electrons results in electrical currents, light, radio waves, and other phenomena.
- **Cell**: the smallest structural unit of living matter capable of functioning independently, consisting of cytoplasm and a nucleus, enclosed by a membrane — the stuff man is made of.

These simple definitions are all that are needed to understand some of the basic concepts; it doesn't take a degree in nuclear physics or cellular biology.

Science tells us that everything in the universe is comprised of spinning particles of light and energy. Everything we touch, taste, see and hear, are made up of these particles. Even the things we can't touch, the things we can't see but yet believe to exist are made up of these particles, including the air we breathe.

Breath isn't just some sort of airy "nothing," it is a particle substance. It is made of air particles, the same as those particles that constitute a spinach quiche, Mt. Rushmore, the planet Jupiter, the Pacific Ocean, the human stomach, or someone's Aunt Natalie somewhere in mid-Missouri. Everything is comprised of particles, and it is the interaction between particles of various molecular and atomic structures that supports form and maintains life. Everything is made of spinning particles of light and energy — *everything.*

What happens when two recognizable objects, like a stomach and a quiche, collide? Well, if the quiche happens to be inside the stomach, other molecules that make up the acids and enzymes of the digestive fluid come into play. The quiche is broken down into its constituent parts — fats, sugars, fibers, mineral, vitamins, etc. The lining of the digestive system is studded with a variety of molecules designed to interact with specific groups of food molecules. These receptor molecules will latch on to the specific fats, sugars, or whatever they were designed to catch, pass them through the lining and into the circulatory system to be carried throughout the entire body. At the end of the line, the molecules that used to be a quiche will interact with the molecules that make up the cells that make up the tissues that make up the organs that make up the body. There they will be taken apart. Their physical constituents and the energy stored in the molecular bonds will be harvested to provide material and energy for the growth and maintenance of the body. It is this process of digestion that makes possible the controlled exchange of energy from one molecule to another for the nourishment of the body, promoting the well-being and healthy development of a specific, living thing.

Hang in there, I'm getting to the yoga bit.

There are a huge variety of substances composed in such a way that they can be consumed and digested to provide nutrition.

Quiche, prunes, yogurt, kale, stir-fry, legumes, fish — anything that is made of the appropriately combined energy particles — is potential nourishment for the body.

If everything is made of the same basic energy particles, why must we think only in terms of physical food as being our sole source of nourishment? If air is nothing more than spinning molecules of light and energy, why can't air be considered as a food for the body? When we breathe, are we not "eating" air? Don't the air molecules move through the walls of the lungs similar to the way the quiche molecules move through the walls of the stomach and intestines? Is it not essentially the same process?

There have been reports throughout history and from many cultures, of individuals — yogins especially — advanced in a lifelong practice of physical and spiritual discipline who fast, existing on little to no food for many days or even weeks with no ill effects. What is it that keeps these people alive? The answer (apparently): they breathe in their nourishment — they "eat" air — and they are as full as if they had eaten an eight-course meal. The way they breathe lets their bodies make use of the maximum amount of energy the air has to offer.

A word about fasting — a disclaimer:

People have engaged in fasting as a spiritual exercise for millennia, and continue to do so today. In recent years fasting for the purpose of enhancing one's health has become quite popular. Modern science has documented many beneficial effects of short-term, intermittent, and even long-term (up to two or three weeks) fasting. These effects can include weight loss (of course) and more efficient metabolism, and there are many case studies of individuals who have experienced control over and even remission of various autoimmune conditions and cancer. Equally well documented are the detrimental effects of extreme and long-term fasting, including dehydration and starvation leading to permanent physical damage and death. A quick search of the internet will turn up dozens to hundreds of blogs, forums, and assorted gurus discussing, promoting, or even selling the latest product, program, or system for fasting the "right" way. The most extreme—and dangerous—of these advocates are those who claim that they have progressed to the level where they have no need to eat any food, ever. These people are frauds and charlatans, and are just plain lying.

Whether for spiritual enhancement or for the health benefit, even a short fast of one or two days requires a certain amount of physical and mental preparation in order to gain the maximum effect. A fast of any longer duration should not be attempted without a medical consultation or even supervision. No fast of any length should be undertaken if you have or suspect you have any medical conditions.

Back to "Eating Air"

The human body is nothing more than a bunch of energy particles, spinning around and bumping into each other. When the energy particles of air are introduced into the human body by inhalation, they join with the body's various energy particles, adding to the energy already present within the body. As you eat food to nourish your body, you also eat air for the same purpose. Breakfast, lunch and dinner provide the correct and proper forms of food we eat, and yoga provides the correct and proper form of air we eat.

These days, without yoga human beings do not get enough air in the course of a normal waking day to provide sufficient nourishment for their bodies. Humans have gotten lazy. Inactivity in a technological society allows people to get by on shallow, short breaths that supply just enough air to get by on.

Most people aren't aware of the expansion and contraction of their lungs with every inhalation and exhalation, and are even less aware of the muscular and skeletal activity required for the process. As an involuntary physical action, it is taken for granted and ignored rather than regarded as the sacred gift from God that it is.

99% of the population doesn't know how to breathe correctly—how to eat enough air to provide for a well-maintained body. Humans tend to breathe through the front of their noses as if they are sniffing an offensive odor. Even when engaged in aerobic activity or a workout at the gym they tend to pant and sniff.

They don't breathe properly. They don't eat air.

Yogins eat air. It has been shown that a serious yogin eats more air in the course of a one-hour yoga session, than an ordinary person does in three days. This is not hard to believe, given the breathing techniques one practices during a normal Yoga class. In a nutshell, the more air a yogin eats, the more balanced and nourished the body will become. You will find instructions for spinal breathing at the end of Chapter 6, "Silence, Prayer, and Meditation." I teach this technique in my workshops and classes, and have used it daily myself for many years.

One should bring to the practice of yoga the same attitude one has in anticipation of a fine dining experience. Yoga isn't just a physical workout or an art form, it is a source of life. In order for it to work, you must take it seriously and do it on a regular basis. In all of my experience as a yogin and a yoga instructor, the main problem I have noticed is that many students simply don't give the process enough time. There are those who come to class once a month and complain that it isn't working for them, and those who come to class three times a week for two weeks then drop out because they claim yoga isn't doing the job. But the problem isn't the yoga. The problem is in the lack of commitment to a yogic lifestyle.

Yoga isn't something you do on a whim for a couple of weeks, like some popular fad diet or exercise. Yoga is a life-long dedication. Yoga isn't something you do only when you go to a class. It is something you must take home with you. It is something you must integrate into your concept of who you are, and this integration comes with commitment to the process. Only then can you expect to find the healing that yoga inevitably leads to.

Take care not to be fooled by trendy yoga. Yoga is more than listening to New Age music while trying to copy the moves of the skinny guy up front in a black outfit who is twisting himself into impossible poses. Yoga is more than looking cool and hip, or in and groovy. Yoga is a formula that works. It is a tried and true method for health and well-being, dating back at least 6,000 years. Just as the formula 2+2=4 each and every time, so does the formula YOGA = health and vitality — every time.

There are many parts to the yogic formula, but they are not complicated or difficult to understand. Take diet, for instance ...

OK, I know you're thinking, "You mean I have to give up meat?"

The answer is NO, but holy cow, consider what you could give up instead. How about your health? It is a fact that many debilitating and fatal diseases such as cancer, heart disease, and diabetes have a possible link to the over-consumption of meat and meat products; not so much the meat itself but the chemicals used in production and processing.

Many yogins are vegetarians not for reasons of health, but because of their own understanding of yogic principles (see *Ahimsa*, the first yogic yama, in Chapter 4). But even among those who adhere to strict abstinence from meat, there is broad acceptance and support of those who choose to eat meat. The key is not so much *what* you eat, but *how* you eat.

If in your journey on the yogic path, you find yourself moved to give up meat, don't be afraid to do so; listen to your body and your spirit. Also realize that being a vegetarian is not a prerequisite for being a yogin. In my experience, I have found that vegetarians are not in the majority among yogins; meat eaters (or rather, omnivores) are, particularly here in the Western world. What does predominate, are people of both persuasions who are eating healthy and healthful food in moderation. They have developed an awareness of the nutrient value of everything they consume, and a respectful regard for where their food came from and for the processes that brought it to their plate.

Other parts of the yogic formula include the principles of yama and niyama (see Chapter 4), meditation or prayer (the quest for some sort of communion with God, Chapter 6), asanas (Chapter 7) and pranayama, or breathing techniques (Chapter 6), and most importantly, the mental and spiritual orientation of a yogin—how does a yogin relate to this world? Just what is this yogic lifestyle all about? What is the purpose of life? Those questions will be answered—or at least discussed further—as you read along.

But back to the breath. Why is proper breathing so important? You say, "I breathe okay. I'm not dead am I?"

Well, you may not be dead, but are you healthy? How do you feel? Are you energetic? Do you have any of those so-called adult-onset diseases? And most importantly, even though you aren't dead yet, is your quality of life what you would like it to be? Your attunement to — that is, your conscious awareness and control of — your breath will determine this and will contribute to increased longevity and quality of life. So don't be like everybody else.

America is a nation of shallow breathers — and the rest of the world doesn't do so well either. It has been shown that the average human being, regardless of where they live, uses only about one third of their lung capacity under normal circumstances. Granted, our lungs are over-engineered just in case we find ourselves running to escape from a lion or to rescue a child from a burning building — neither being situations faced by many of us every day. The relatively sedate and sedentary nature of normal modern life allows the air in the deep recess of our lungs to stagnate, and the muscles and tissues that facilitate deep breathing to stiffen and atrophy. Proper yogic breathing can keep the entirety of your lungs functioning properly and with full reserve capacity when you need it.

Your body is like your house. When all the windows are closed there is still plenty of air to breathe, but after awhile it gets stale. When you open the windows on a fine day, a fresh breeze comes in and sweeps out the accumulated odors of daily living. Often it is not until the new air has replaced the old air that you realize just how bad things had gotten. After years of unconscious shallow breathing your body begins to suffer. It's not noticeable at first, but over time the lack of oxygen begins to leave its mark on your body, mind, and emotions. A lack of oxygen effects the function of your organs (heart, liver, kidneys, etc.), speeds up the aging process, and increases the long-term possibility for the development of those adult-onset diseases such as asthma, diabetes, high blood pressure, Alzheimer's, depression, etc. They are most likely the result of, and are certainly exacerbated by, years of improper breathing. Bad things happen when the brain and body are starved of oxygen. It is logical to assume that these diseases that creep up on us, and of which we are not aware until we are firmly in their grip, are the result of, or are accelerated by that starvation, as there is considerable research to substantiate this conclusion.

The brain is the control center for everything you are and everything you do. If the brain is starved of oxygen its control over the systems of the body will be disturbed and might even fail completely. It has even been shown that when the brain is starved of oxygen, alterations occur in the regions controlling human emotion. If you are experiencing depression, PTSD, or any kind of emotional trauma, your may find relief by simply signing up for a local yoga class. Even simpler, develop your own daily routine of the postures given in this book, as they have all been selected specifically for (among other things) their abilities to heal many of the problems caused by poor breathing. Practice the postures—every day, if possible—for three months, and see if you are not changed for the better.

You can be eating the healthiest food on this planet, but if you are not breathing correctly, it won't matter what you eat. The processes of ingesting, digesting, and assimilating food are only part of the cycle; it is oxygen that provides the energy required to keep the fire of life burning within the cells of your body. The food you eat can't be broken down and properly incorporated and used by your physical system unless you breathe correctly. The molecular processes that are designed to bring nourishment and healing down inside the digestive tract can't do it, because the element of oxygen is not present in its necessary, required amount. We need to take in—to *ingest* air—in order to get the job done.

The intake of air and food is only half of the process of eating and breathing. Once the components of the food you have eaten interact at the cellular level with the oxygen you have breathed, and all the good parts have been incorporated and the energy put to use, there are waste products to be collected and removed. It is the second part of breathing—the exhale—that is instrumental in this process.

Ineffective breathing not only restricts the amount of oxygen entering your body, it also impedes the removal of toxins from your body, resulting in weakness and ill health, in both body and mind.

And when you don't feel good, you are less likely to be concerned with the spiritual aspects of your life, which are also crucial in maintaining health and well-being on several levels of your journey to self-discovery.

As you age, your body's processes and functions begin to deteriorate, and fall short of what they were when you were a teenager. Your tissues and organs harden and shrink, becoming inefficient in their exchange of oxygen and toxins. It is necessary to increase the amount of oxygen you are able to consume as you grow older. The good thing is that every technique for increasing oxygen intake results in an equal increase of waste removal. Unfortunately, the opposite usually occurs. As humans age, their activity tends to decrease, leading in turn to a reduction in oxygen intake and an increase in toxin retention. The final result is that they literally begin to die of starvation and poison. It has been demonstrated that the more air you breathe the more energy you retain, even into so-called old age.

Remember, old age has little to do with the number of years you have dwelt on this planet. It has to do with the way you have taken care of yourself. Old age sneaks up on you as a result of bad habits, improper nutrition, and lack of oxygen. Sure, genetics has a lot to do with it, but even genetics can be detoured by a dedication to the life-giving practice of yoga. Over the years I have personally known many people who had been given a death sentence by their own genetic history. Much of that was reversed after attending yoga classes for only a few months. I've kept in contact with many of those same individuals who have now lived years past the time the doctors had told them to expect to pass on to that "great Ashram in the sky".

Of course, those students were serious about changing their destinies, and they chose to adopt the yogic lifestyle as the best way to accomplish that goal. These people did not come to a class just once in a while. They attended regularly and took seriously all of the advice and instruction given in those classes and which form the basis of this book.

Thousands of years ago a group of yogins gathered together certain precepts, codes, and practices that they held in common. Adding some personal thoughts and preferences, they organized them into what we know today as yoga. They didn't know it at the time, but they were developing the first scientific system for the enhancement of health and quality of life. When you begin to practice the postures, the breathing, the diet, and the other yogic principles, some of the first changes you notice are improved flexibility, renewed strength, a slimmer body, improved posture and balance, clearer thought processes, and heightened stamina, just to name a few. These obvious changes are wonderful and encouraging, but there are more changes going on inside the body without even being aware of them.

Yoga stimulates a gradual molecular change deep inside that will eventually alter your desires, as well as the way you look at and relate to the world around you. "You are what you eat" is, indeed, a true statement. If you eat a lot of meat, fat, and sugar you will become obese and unhealthy. If you eat a lot of healthy vegetables, fruit, and lean meats in moderation, you will become lean and healthy.

The same is true on the metaphysical plane. If you *EAT YOGA!* you will become yogic, which implies not just physical changes but spiritual changes as well. After practicing yoga for only three months—sincerely practicing it—you will find yourself to be a totally different person. You may not even recognize the new you.

It has been a pleasure over the years to watch as my students have evolved from one state of existence to another over relatively short periods of time. I have students who were in their 70s and even 80s, who grew up in the Midwest consuming great hunks of sausage, red meat, and fried chicken, with that greasy white-flour gravy that always accompanies fried chicken. They consumed pork roasts, ham, bacon, eggs and fried potatoes by the tons. I watched them shed all of those things that they were once so fond of after just a few months of yoga practice. Every one of those students made radical changes to their diets, some even became vegetarians. Their health changed. Their complexion changed. Their stamina changed. Everything about them changed for the better.

They became yogins! And they loved it. They loved it because they lost weight, lowered their high blood pressure, their cholesterol plummeted, their breathing improved, their arthritis disappeared, and more importantly, their entire outlook on life completely changed. Many had gone from an attitude of bitterness and defeatism, to one of positive and energetic hope. Some had even feared death to such an extent that they almost gave up on living, but their commitment to the yogic lifestyle altered them to such a degree that they didn't even think about death any more. They didn't fear it because the yogic lifestyle taught them that even death holds no power over anyone; that death is only a very short passage to the next great adventure in eternal life. Remember that in your true, eternal form, you are a spirit, and your spirit is made of energy, and energy never dies. You just change form when you float up out of that flesh body at the moment humans call death.

Yoga changes everyone who adopts it as a lifestyle into peaceful, healthy beings, and much of the change can be linked to proper breathing. Studies have shown that juvenile delinquency and adult criminal behavior are aggravated by shallow breathing. Teenagers with serious tendencies toward violence and disciplinary problems who have been enrolled in yoga programs have shown dramatic improvements in behavior. Hardened criminals who used to carry guns and knives and rob liquor stores are living normal lives, raising families, and working at full time jobs after three or four months of regular yoga practice.

And that isn't all. The latest research shows that yoga can be instrumental in slowing, and in some cases even halting, the progression of Alzheimer's disease, memory loss, dementia, and many other maladies of aging. I have had more than one doctor tell me that they were convinced that the primary reason for the improvement of brain disorders such as these was the breathing techniques taught in some yoga classes.

It's all in the breath that is intrinsically interwoven with the asanas, and the diet, and the entire lifestyle of being a yogin. It is gratifying to see progress made in the lives of people who had decided years ago to give life one more chance and try yoga.

We are what we eat. If you *EAT YOGA!* you will reap the benefits. You will no longer be troubled by the world around you, you will no longer allow the silly little things in life to upset you, you will be physically strong, you will be mentally alert, and you will be spiritually fulfilled.

You must, however, take yoga seriously. You should attend a professional class as least once each week, making sure that it is taught by a fully certified yoga instructor who lives the lifestyle, and doesn't just play the pretty music while continually interrupting the class with nonsensical chatter.

Be aware that there are a lot of yoga styles and teachers out there, and it does make a difference which one you choose. I advise you to select a gentle yoga class that allows you the freedom to change the rigidity of a posture in order to meet the needs of your own body.

There are commercial franchises that have reduced yoga to an ego-driven sport, focusing on an unnatural physical perfection of posture and form, while paying little attention to specific needs, motivation, and limitations of the student. When you go into a yoga class for the first time and you see only young people with perfect bodies sweating and grunting and strutting around like movie stars, turn around and run for your life.

Choose instead an independent teacher who is gentle and understanding, and who can offer suggestions on how to make the class easier for you while guiding your progress forward. Just because a yoga teacher is cute, young, and bubbly, does not mean he or she will be the right fit for you. Shop around. Smaller classes are better than larger classes. Quiet, non-aggressive teachers are better than loud, boisterous teachers with sexy outfits and microphones hanging around their necks. Find an experienced teacher who has tailored his or her class around the health needs of the students and not the fads and fashions of the contemporary yoga market.

There is something special about being in a yoga class with other students. There is an energy that is not present when you are doing yoga alone at home. Everything you need for living a yogic lifestyle is in this book, but if you are serious about your health and wellbeing, attending a class with like-minded individuals will enhance your efforts.

Some Final Thoughts

You must make a sincere effort to practice the asanas and the breathing techniques in your own home, as often as you can. You must attempt to live your life in a way that will bring no harm to others or to yourself.

Follow the dietary principles of yoga as much as possible. Remember, you are not required to be a vegetarian. To paraphrase the advice given by Paramhansa Yogananda:

Being a vegetarian is a good thing, but it is not necessary for the salvation of a human soul. If that were so, then none of the Eskimos up north could attain salvation because they depend almost totally upon animal flesh and fat for their very existence.

Above all, it is not the food you eat that is important, but the spirit in which it was acquired, prepared and consumed.

4

Principles to Live By

No book about yoga would be complete without an examination of yama and niyama, the "don'ts and do's" of yoga. These are sometimes referred to as the Ten Commandments of Yoga, but don't let that bother you; they have little to do with organized religion. Moving past the Hindu designations, you will find that these core principles are simple and easy to follow; mostly just plain old common sense. Read slowly and consider each point carefully, envisioning how you can incorporate them into your own sphere of existence.

Yamas

The yama principles are the restraints — the "don'ts". Each of the five listed here are actions and attitudes over which one must learn to exercise control or even abstinence. These are the things that weigh you down and bring turmoil to your lives, filling you with discontent, and worse, making you feel guilty about seeking God.

Ahimsa: Don't bring harm to any living creature, including to yourself.

It is no accident that this yama, which translates as non-violence, non-injury, and harmlessness, is listed first. Everything that can be done should be done before resorting to violence of any kind, and then, don't do it! If one can gain mastery over one's inclination to lash out — either in aggression or defense — then adherence to all of the other principles will follow. This quality is demonstrated to the highest degree in the life and teachings of Mohandas Gandhi. He made his personal commitment to the principles of nonviolence public, first in South Africa, then more notably in India. There are many biographies of this great man, but my favorite is *Gandhi An Autobiography: The Story Of My Experiments With Truth*. I highly recommend it as an interesting read and as a source of inspiration.

Make ahimsa a part of your very being, like breathing itself. We are confronted everyday with challenges to our inner tranquility. At work, for instance: your co-worker is awarded that promotion you worked so hard to get. You know you deserve it much more than he does! You worked twice as long and twice as hard as he did, but the boss apparently likes his suits better than yours (or something like that) and he got the job. You smile and say, "Congratulations," but you are seething inside. You've never hit another person in your life, but ...

Ahimsa instructs that you are not even supposed to think violent thoughts. To carry out violence is a bad thing, but to imagine violence in your heart and mind is as bad. Just as words have power behind them, so do thoughts. Negative thoughts—even when repressed—can be displayed in your physical actions, causing more conflict and turmoil around you. On the other hand, positive thoughts can lead to positive actions, which can actually bring healing to situations that were bad in the beginning. People who think good things are almost always good on the outside, and goodness is a great way to strengthen your bond with God and all those around you. So, take control of your mind. Congratulate and bless your co-worker not just with your lips, but from your heart as well.

If you are serious about becoming a true yogin, ahimsa means to remove all violence from your life. That means hunting and fishing just for fun, attending certain sporting events or watching them on TV, violent movies, road rage, cursing people under your breath—you get the picture.

The principle of ahimsa is a difficult one to live by, as our current culture is prone to violence and displays of aggression, even in our recreational activities. When you first begin to practice it, you may find yourself separated or isolated from people you had considered to be your friends. But as you progress along the yogic path you will begin to question many of your past practices, and you will not be able to justify or rationalize retaining them, as you enter a new life of peace—ahimsa.

Satya: Don't lie

This one should be pretty easy to comprehend. It means exactly what it says: DON'T LIE. We are, of course, speaking of things of a serious nature. Sometimes it is permissible to conceal certain information in order to protect either a person or a greater need for humanity. Sometimes it may be necessary to embellish the facts in order to do the same. Strict adherence to facts is not the same thing as being truthful. You must be the judge of those instances for your own life. Remember, everything comes down to the attitude of the heart when it comes to justifying any word or deed. If you must err, do so on the side of compassion. And, yes, it is okay to stretch the truth in silly things any time you are playing with your children; that is called, having fun. But never lie intentionally in order to selfishly advance your own interests or to bring harm to someone.

Ashteya: Don't steal

Are these yogic principles beginning to look familiar? *"Thou shalt not steal."* (Deuteronomy 5:19) Again, it is hard to miss the meaning of this one. It's simple and to the point. Don't take anything that isn't yours to take. If it belongs to someone else, it's not yours. That means taking paper clips from work, a wallet you find on the street, cheating on your income tax, borrowing a shovel from a neighbor and never returning it, or robbing a bank. In the eyes of God they're all the same, and God's eyes see everything. You may be able to hide that shovel from your neighbor, but you can't hide it from God.

It's easy to see how ashteya relates to items that have a physical presence, but it can relate to intangibles as well. How many times have you provided a listening ear or a shoulder to cry on for someone needing advice or comfort and found yourself thinking about how you can make yourself seem smarter, more important, or even indispensable, rather than truly listening to the other person? By not giving the other person your full and selfless attention, you are stealing their time and preying on their need, which is every bit as bad as—or worse than—stealing their wallet.

Brahmacharya: Don't waste your energy

Brahmacharya is most often thought of in terms of practicing non-sensuality, as in to control or restrict sexuality—practicing celibacy outside of marriage and fidelity within a marriage. As such, it tends to get less consideration in our modern and "enlightened" society than it should. To get a better understanding of this guiding principle substitute "sensuality" for "sexuality". "Sensuality" in this context means to be overly devoted to the pleasures of the senses.

How often have you been distracted by the sight of a hot new sports car, and felt a bit of material lust in your heart while your budget is telling you to stick with the Dodge Neon? How about that gorgeous dress that was way too expensive but you bought it any way, and you only wore it once? Or what about that big new house of yours that you can barely make the payments on, but it has the most luxurious bathroom ever? These indulgences in sensual pleasures create mental and emotional turmoil and divert your energies away from the attainment of peace and tranquility in your life.

How about the sense of hearing? How do you break the principle of brahmacharya with that one? Well, there was that dirty joke someone told at work on Friday. You listened to it and laughed right along with everybody else. And wasn't that a juicy bit of gossip you heard in church last Sunday? Bet you can't wait to pass it on to someone else.

Gossip is one of the most harmful and destructive forces known to humanity. It has ruined more friendships, destroyed more relationships, hurt more feelings, than just about anything I can think of. It is a terrible thing and it has no part in the yogic lifestyle. If someone attempts to feed you a juicy line about someone else, shut it down if you can. Try to set the record straight, or at least walk away from it. Moreover, in the quiet of your own mind, direct loving thoughts toward the victim. You will be energetically assisting all those involved, including the one doing the harmful talk. Remember also that 99% of all gossip is untrue, exaggerated, and *always* with evil intent. Just don't go there.

The ears are the portals for much of what diverts our

spiritual energy. How many of you listen to the news each day and let yourself get upset and agitated about things beyond your control? It seems like things get worse every day, and yet you can't pull yourself away from it. In addition, we are subjected to ever-increasing amounts of noise in our environment. These noises are frequencies that interfere with, obscure, or destroy the vital frequencies of Creation that we depend on for our life and health, both physical and spiritual. Take care in choosing what you listen to.

Probably the most tempting sensual pleasure is the pleasure of food—the taste, the textures, and the aroma beguile our senses and entice us to over indulge. According to the latest studies, 70% of Americans are now overweight and about 37% are downright obese. This is a shame, and much of it is simply because humans choose to exercise very little self-discipline over their lives. They sit in front of their computers and televisions, chomping their chips, and chowing down anything, and everything, within reach—the greasier, the sweeter, or the saltier, the better.

The food industry is indeed responsible for some of the problem by producing products that cater to our taste for more sugar, fat, and salt, and that will be converted to fat and poison in the human system. The biggest blame though, rests solidly on the shoulders of the consumer. Humans are fat because they choose to be fat. They are destroying their health because they choose to do so. No one follows them around all day forcing them to eat junk food, drink diet sodas, and binge on alcoholic beverages—the most concentrated form of empty calories a person can consume.

Self-control is something that humans have trouble with, especially when it comes to food. Part of the problem is that people often feel restless, dissatisfied, or unhappy, but can't figure out why or what to do about it. Food provides immediate gratification and distraction from the ongoing problems in one's life. Chocolate for instance, has been proven to be almost as effective as certain drugs as a mood elevator. And what about "comfort food", those fat-laden and carbohydrate-rich dishes from childhood that make us feel better when we're feeling sorry for ourselves? And what is better when you are feeling restless or fidgety than a bag of crunchy, salty, greasy chips? I'm not saying that these things are not to be enjoyed occasionally or in moderation, but if you find yourself over indulging on a regular basis, you might be guilty of wasting your energies on avoidance of the real issue.

Proper weight control is one result of following the principle of brahmacharya. If you have difficulty in this area, don't lose heart. By following the yogic lifestyle as presented here, your body will soon adjust to a weight that is ideal for your health and wellbeing. Yoga is directional; it begins at where you are right now and takes you forward, not backward. You may be breaking all of the principles of brahmacharya right now, but you've only just started on the path. Give it a few weeks and see what happens.

Even your desire to satisfy your sense of touch can get you into trouble. When you were just a child your Mother told you not to touch that hot pan—you did anyway. The little girl who sat in front of you in the third grade had a thick ponytail that just begged to be pulled. How did that work out for you?

Years ago I used to haunt the art museums in Los Angeles. Every once in a while I would come across a painting or sculpture that just cried out for me to touch it—just one quick touch to connect with the artist for one brief moment. Museums have strict rules about touching the art, and with good reason, but ... Well, I did, and I got caught. The guard took pity on me and let me off with a warning. There could have been serious consequences, such as being banished from the museum. Since then, I have exercised control over that particular impulse.

By practicing the principle of brahmacharya—self-control— you will find your life becoming less chaotic and more ordered. You will be able to focus your energy toward filling your life with peace and tranquility and spiritual growth.

Aparigraha: Don't be greedy

Greed can be defined as the intense and insatiable craving for things such as wealth, possessions, food, and power. Just as brahmacharya is self-control over one's body, aparigraha is self-control over one's desires.

Greed is like cancer. It grows inside you, starting off as a tiny thing you don't even know you have, then spreads to infect every area of your life until one day you can't get rid of it. You can't get enough wealth. You can't get enough property. You can't get enough power. You can't get enough cake.

Almost every terrible thing you can think of that is happening in the world today, as far as countries getting along with each other, can be traced back to greed—one country wanting something that another country has. How many wars have been driven by this terrible disease throughout the centuries? Not just big wars either, but little spats over boundaries, grazing rights, water rights, and stray cattle. All fueled by greed—the unyielding desire to get something or to keep something. It is easy to identify the consequences of greed in the events of the world and society we live in, but greed is a cause of turmoil and conflict in the lives and inner beings of individuals, as well.

At the heart of the principle of aparigraha, is the ability to recognize sufficiency. Did you wake up in a bed this morning and with a roof over your head? Do you have clothing and shoes? Have you eaten today? Be grateful to have the basic needs of your life met. Enjoy the things you have, but don't become attached to them. Don't waste your energy and resources on the desire for more, bigger, better, newer, or more luxurious. Focus instead on what is necessary for your own yogic path. When you get right down to it, material things are just "stuff." And just how much stuff does a yogin need?

The word *yama* may be foreign to the English-speaking world, but the principles of yama are not. This country was founded on many of these same spiritual tenets. Some are even written into the Constitution, as well as the Bill of Rights, yet how many Americans conscientiously apply these ideals to their lives? This inherent and expected system of ethics and morals lies at the very heart of yoga, and must be put into practice if you truly wish to claim this lifestyle that dates back to the beginning of recorded history.

Niyamas

Where the yamas are the guiding principles for your relationship with and conduct toward the world outside of yourself, the niyamas are the guides to how you should treat yourself, physically and spiritually.

If the word "don't" is hard for you to handle, then focus on the niyamas first. By cultivating the actions and attitudes prescribed by these principles, you will find yourself changing from the inside out and falling into adherence to the yamas with little or no effort.

Correct practice of these principles is truly transformational, molding you into what you are meant to be and keeping you on your yogic path for a lifetime.

Saucha: Practice cleanliness and purity.

Many of the practices and general principles of yoga are directed toward purification of the body, mind, and spirit, so it is no wonder that the principle of saucha is listed first, as it covers so much of the yogic goal of ultimate wellbeing.

These days, it is universally acknowledged that a certain level of cleanliness about one's body and surroundings, and purity of one's food and water is required to maintain health, or in some situations, even to survive. Likewise, a certain level of mental and spiritual cleanliness and order is essential if one is to achieve a healthy mind and an enlightened soul.

The concept of mental cleanliness must not be ignored or taken lightly. A cluttered, undisciplined mind interferes with the flow of energy between body, soul, and mind, resulting in a loss of purpose or sense of identity, and in a physical and spiritual malaise, a condition underlying many forms of disease — or dis-ease — physical, mental, and spiritual.

According to the Lore of the Internet — in itself a source of mental clutter — the human brain produces 70,000 thoughts per day, give or take a few. While scientific verification of this number seems to be completely lacking, and there seems to be wide disagreement about what actually constitutes a discreet thought, there can be no argument that human brains are very active on both the conscious and subconscious levels.

The issue is quality, not quantity. How can you not think some bad thoughts once in a while? When I say "bad thoughts," I don't necessarily mean evil scenarios, plots, and schemes. I mean undisciplined thoughts, like those that enter your consciousness and distract you from the task you need to complete; or the thoughts that arise when a few words of conversation pull you away from the present, depriving a friend of your attention and support at a critical time; or the worst—those thoughts that bubble up in the quiet moments just before sleep or meditation, calling attention to all of your past transgressions, real or imagined, and eroding your very sense of self—your mind, soul, and spirit.

This kind of mental and emotional negativity can be addictive. The feelings of rage, hatred, anger, jealousy, lust, greed, doubt, etc., produce physiological responses, which, if left unchecked, damage the body and cause physical debilitation and disease.

The principle of saucha asks that you make every effort to control your thoughts, and if you are striving for the purity that is the essence of the yogic lifestyle, you must make every attempt to rid your mind of any thought that will lead you from the path. It is difficult, but the words of the Apostle Paul give encouragement:

> *"Finally brethren, whatsoever things are true, whatsoever things are honest, whatsoever things are just, whatsoever things are pure, whatsoever things are lovely, whatsoever things are of good report, if there be any virtue, and if there be any praise, think on these things."*
> (Philippians 4:8)

Recollection of Paul's advice can break the cycle of negativity and impurity and allow physical and spiritual healing to begin. What would this world be like if everyone took these words to heart?

How do we maintain the discipline of a pure body, mind, and spirit if we are surrounded by forces that would drag us into the mud? First of all, our choice of friends can make all the difference.

As a middle school administrator, it was among my duties

to monitor the behavior of the students, particularly the youngest as they made the transition from the more protective and orderly elementary school environment in which a single teacher was the primary influence in a single classroom. The middle school, by contrast, was a more chaotic environment. Instead of a single teacher teaching multiple subjects in a single classroom, the students moved between multiple classrooms where each teacher was dedicated to teaching a single subject. The passing periods, along with extended opportunities for before and after school activities allowed ample time for the young students to practice their budding social skills among their peers. We expect children to change rapidly as they move from elementary to middle school — it's called growing up — but we want them to grow up as themselves, not as little reflections of popular culture. The pressure to be like everyone else at that age is tremendous, and very often even the best of kids begin to talk, walk, dress, and otherwise behave like their more charismatic and less virtuous contemporaries, questioning or abandoning the morals and values of their parents while adopting those of their peers and their pop icons without reservation.

As one emerges on the adult side of adolescence, it is to be hoped that one has gained the confidence to make life choices based on the knowledge of an eternal and infinite existence beyond this physical world. Even so, decent people often get caught up with companions and entangled in situations that cause them to loose site of their true values. These behaviors and associations may be of apparent benefit in the short term, but the long-term effect is loss of moral grounding, alienation of true friends and loved ones, increased stress and illness, depression, and dissatisfaction with life. A mind that is weakened in this way will seek comfort and justification in shallow, worldly relationships that feed only the ego and not the spirit, dragging one further into darkness and away from the Light.

The writings of Paramhansa Yogananda are filled with his expressions of concern regarding one's choice of companions:

"There is a constant change of magnetism between you and your surroundings and the people with whom you come in contact ... all actions, both positive and negative, create vibrations in the ether. These vibrations are everywhere present. When you are in the environment of these vibrations, they pass through your body just like radio waves. If you live or associate with people who are doing wrong, you will feel the magnetic vibration of their wrongdoing, no matter how you try to avoid it. Weak-minded individuals should by all means shun the company of those with bad habits."
(The Divine Romance)

This sentiment is repeated throughout Yogananda's books and essays, giving clear warning to everyone that all negative people are to be avoided. If you find yourself in the company of someone shedding negative energies like cat hair, just turn your back and leave. If you find that your current situation or relationship is interfering with your spiritual growth, then it is time for a change.

Chapter 9 of the Book of Luke begins with the instructions that Jesus gave to the twelve disciples as He sent them out to preach His message of peace and to heal the sick. As much as Jesus wanted all the world to understand and to adopt His peaceful teachings, His final instruction was this:

If people do not welcome you, leave their town and shake the dust off your feet as a testimony against them.
Luke 9:5 (NIV)

In other words, if the disciples were not well-received, or if they were abused in any way as they presented His Truths, they were to shun those who were working against them, and move on. He did not ask them to take reprisal for bad treatment, or to punish anyone just because they did not adopt His Teachings. He did tell His disciples to move on, leave those people to their own devices, and find others who would be more receptive.

Simply put, Saucha is a concern for the whole person—inside and out—and for the environment one chooses for oneself. It goes beyond clean body and clean mind; it envelops the metaphysical world of everything and everyone you come into contact with. Every thought, every deed, every person, every place, every experience, every entertainment, and every diversion—all are to be governed by a sense of Saucha.

Santosha: Practice contentment

The niyama of santosha compliments the yamas of brahmacharya (non-sensuality) and aparigraha (non-greed.) People who are greedy or who live for the senses are never content with what they have. Each acquisition leads to the desire for more, and each sensual experience leaves a craving for greater intensity. When one practices contentment, the urges to possess material things and to gratify the senses are put into their proper perspectives. True santosha—true contentment—is perhaps the greatest virtue and the greatest gift of the yogic lifestyle. The serious yogin knows that there is nothing more to acquire than that which is already possessed. The yogin is content because happiness is not found in cars, or boats, or jewelry, or music, or sports, or religion, or positions of power, but in inner peace and in a relationship with God. Contentment is the bliss that is felt with the first connection a person makes with the Divine Creator of the Universe. Santosha is understood when simplicity is combined with fulfillment and acceptance. It is another facet of God's Peace. The Creator promises that commitment to a lifestyle such as that suggested here in these pages, will lead to the understanding that santosha is a link to the Divine energy not found in the things of this world.

Tapas: Practice discipline

One of the first things a person does after deciding to "get into" yoga is buy a yoga mat. The first mats designed and produced specifically for the practice of yoga were given the trademarked name of Tapas. Over the years, other companies have produced mats with various properties and of differing quality, and given them clever names, but yoga practitioners tend to refer to them generically as "tapas mats"—kind of like calling all fizzy cola drinks "coke". All yogic teachings and practices are intended to bring discipline and focus to one's life. The principle of tapas defines and describes that focus, and it is on the mat that the aspiring yogin engages in the physical disciplines of the asanas while contemplating the mental and spiritual disciplines of the yamas and niyamas.

Every serious practitioner of yoga must learn discipline in all things that are yogic—the asanas, diet, meditation and prayer, yama, niyama, breathing—because it is their totality that comprise the spiritual science of yoga. These things must not be just added to your life, but incorporated into it. These practices must become as natural as getting up and putting your pants on in the morning. Make them a priority in your life so that your life becomes centered on the practice of yoga, and all other things—your job, your marriage, your family—will fall into place.

The key is to interweave the science and philosophy of yoga into your daily living. Take the yogic mentality to work with you; you will do a far better job and your co-workers will respect you more and, perhaps, be drawn to you for help and advice. They will see something in your demeanor and countenance, something about your smile or your eyes that will suggest to them that you are not like all the others who waste their energy on the frivolous distractions of our superficial, materialistic culture.

Apply yoga to your family. Every principle of the yogic lifestyle centers on harmony and love. How can this do anything but strengthen family relationships?

The philosophy of tapas encourages you to discipline yourself to do everything you can in order to center your being on the practice of pure yoga—to "become" yoga in all that you do and say and think.

Swadhyaya: Practice introspection, or self-study

What do you do when you find yourself with a little free time on your hands? Do you busy yourself with meaningless tasks and endeavors? Do you distract yourself by mindlessly watching the television? What kind of hobbies do you spend your empty hours on? Do you visit bars or other places where people gather for diversion? How many forgettable movies, adolescent football games, or mindless basketball games pass before your eyes? Do you surround yourself with the constant noise of popular music? All of these activities drain our energy and lure us away from the careful observation of our own thoughts, feelings and motivations that must be undertaken before any truly significant changes can take hold in one's life.

This kind of introspection can be daunting to the point of being discouraging, demoralizing, or even frightening. How long has it been since you opened up a spiritual book? If you are a Christian, how long has it been since you opened up the Bible and really took the time to study it? If you are a practitioner of another path, how long has it been since you opened up your books and tried to emulate the founders of your faith? The inspired words of wisdom that comprise the scriptures give guidance and direction to one's personal journey of self-discovery.

The sequence of postures that we commonly refer to as yoga cannot be taken seriously without knowing why you are doing them. You can't really practice the principles of yama and niyama until you first see the necessity for them in your personal sphere of existence. These things can only be discovered by regular and honest introspection accompanied by immersion in a regular study of whatever scriptures you need to further advance yourself on the yogic path.

In every great scripture of every great religion or spiritual path throughout history, there are passages that plead for the disciple to take the scripture seriously — to study it diligently and to apply it personally. Scriptures are more than just ink on paper; they are the very embodiment of the religion or path itself, of all the thoughts and wisdom of all the great masters, gurus, teachers, and apostles. They are the expression and clarification of some of the wisdom that God has been attempting to knock into human heads for thousands of years, and you must take them seriously.

That said, it is best to avoid the commentaries intended to clarify or simplify the original scriptures. Go directly to the source scriptures. Open your heart, and allow them to speak to you personally without any added and questionable opinion as to "what they really mean." When humans add to, or takeaway from the originals, they always distort them, inserting their own personal agendas and rendering the originals powerless and worthless.

Swadhyaya is an absolute necessity for the serious yogin. How can you expect to advance along your path if you remain stagnant in your studies? The more you learn about yoga, the more you will become committed to a lifestyle that will bring increasing health and well-being to your existence.

Find the time to turn off the TV for just an extra half hour each day, and pick up your Bible or Gita, or a book by Yogananda, or Thomas Merton, or a yoga book that is filled with discussions and descriptions of the yogic lifestyle (like this one). How about a gardening magazine to learn how Nature does its thing, or a cookbook for the inspiration to provide healthful and lovingly prepared food? Anything that has anything to do with your newly found path can be considered as material worthy of study. Then take the time to contemplate how your newly acquired knowledge can enhance your spiritual growth. The time spent practicing the physical disciplines of the asanas is an excellent time to practice the intellectual and spiritual discipline of swadhyaya.

Remember, however, that the goal of this type of study when done in the true spirit of swadhyaya is not simply to gain knowledge, but to approach it in such a way as to gain honest knowledge of one's self.

Ishwara Pranidhana: Practice devotion to God

Ishwara is a Sanskrit word that can translate to "Supreme Being", or "God". Pranidhana means "devotion" or "surrender". While it is not within the purview of yoga to provide an explanation of Whom or What God is, it is clear that acknowledgment of and genuine devotion to God, Supreme Being, or Creator is central to the yogic life.

Devotion is not an activity you schedule in your daily planner. It's more than just sitting in church and hearing another variation of the sermon you've heard a thousand times before. It is more than singing a few hymns or bowing your head in prayer or dropping a dollar or two in the collection plate. It is more than burning incense and spinning prayer wheels. Devotion is more than holding up your hands, praising God with your lips, crying crocodile tears, and swaying to the music, only to go home and return to your daily routine with no further thought or reflection.

Devotion is the total immersion of your entire life into the worship of God. You become a walking prayer. Your every thought is a hymn to the Heavens. Your every mannerism, action, deed, and desire, is centered on the teachings that have now become such a part of you that you can no longer imagine life without them. In fact, you have come to realize that life without them is not life at all. A life without devotion is a life of illusion and failure; it is a dead-end existence where the past counts for nothing and the future is hazy at best, and terrifying at worst.

When I became a serious, practicing yogin, I no longer felt obligated to worship God in a regimented, organized way. For me, the need to worship was no longer driven by superstition, it was a yearning, a desire, a heartfelt joy to seek and become close to the God I knew to be near me. My "religion" encompassed everything around me.

In 1 Corinthians 6:19, the Apostle Paul says:

What? Know ye not that your body is the temple of the Holy Spirit which is in you, which ye have of God, and ye are not your own?"

In the Gospel of John, Chapter 17, Jesus prays to God

[21]... that they (you) all be one; as thou, Father, art in me, and I in thee, that they also may be one in us ... [23]I in them, and thou in me, that they may be made perfect in one ...

You carry a piece of God's Spirit and Teachings around with you in your heart and your soul, but it is only when you rid yourself of what does not belong that God can wash through. God is carrying you, and you have only to wake up to that fact. It's not necessary to search for the Presence of God, it's only necessary that you accept the fact that He is already present and you must return to God in full. Once that acceptance and commitment occurs, the devotion comes as naturally as a heartbeat.

With true devotion, you are able to see God in all things. His Presence is the Light you sometimes see glowing in the face of a stranger on the street. You find His Life in every tree or flower, in every animal or rock. God's Presence becomes so strong in your life that devotion to that Presence is no longer something you can turn on and off on certain days or at specific hours. Your devotion now shows clearly in everything you do or say.

If you feel the need to attend a church or fellowship of some kind — socializing with like-minded individuals is often uplifting to your own practice of devotion — find a fellowship that is not at odds with the yogic lifestyle. There are some churches where yoga is looked on with suspicion or disapproval, where it is thought to be "of the devil," but there are many others where yoga is welcomed with understanding. It's not so much a matter of what denomination a church is as it is a matter of who has stolen that church from God and turned it into his or her own little private religion. Jesus never condemned yoga; in fact much of what He did and taught was very similar to what I've written here in this book.

I would love to be able to refer you to a yoga church, but there really aren't any. There are some yoga ashrams (schools) that have their own "churches" attached to them, but they are not readily available to join unless you live near their location. Also, they are often as biased against Christianity as some of the Christians are against yoga, so it wouldn't do you much good to attend in those places.

Yoga styles, techniques, schools, and teaching methods are just as numerous and varied as any of the Christian denominations out there, and in common with those denominations, adherents of each yoga school or style think theirs is the best and all of the others are somehow substandard to the "way it should be." The same can be said for any of the New Age, New Thought styled churches and centers. They, too, are infused with the old egoistic mentality that professes theirs as the best way, and that all the others are off track somehow. Quite frankly, I have felt closer to God and more widely accepted in many Christian churches than I have in yoga centers or schools. Which only goes to prove what I just said, that it isn't what is being taught in a particular location or facility, but how human beings are distorting the teachings, regardless of the religion or philosophy they are selling. If you keep your eyes open and ask around, you will be able to find a church where you will feel welcome and comfortable.

The practice of yoga is mostly a solitary one, however. Remember, yoga means to be yoked, or joined, to God, and I am probably not the first one to tell you that you can't be yoked to church or fellowship and all go to Heaven as a group. Devotion is a personal thing that each one of us must do all on our own.

Your yoga class can be your socialization area. If you have the right teacher, your yoga class can become a spiritual retreat for you, a "church" you can begin with. But remember that it's a "you and God" thing. God is not always found in religions these days, but you can have true church anywhere you and God are together. The Bible teaches that it is the body that is the Temple of the Spirit of God, not the building.

5

A Yogic Guide to Nutrition

Yoga is a lifestyle of moderation and mental clarity, and in this chapter I will give you some basic information to help you apply that concept to your dietary choices. I will also present my own rationale for maintaining a mostly vegetarian diet.

Remember, this book is called "EAT YOGA!" and just as the name implies, yoga is more than just a stretching exercise; it is all about *eating* or *consuming* health as it is derived from proper breathing, exercise, and diet. In effect, these are not things you do to your body, they are things you feed your body. Remember too, that everything is made up of molecules bound together by energy, and it is the interaction of the food, water, and air molecules, and the transfer of energy from those molecules to the molecules of your body that bring you health, longevity, and well-being. In effect, when you practice the yoga postures, breathe properly, and eat a proper diet, you are feeding your body nourishing energy. You are EATING YOGA. Keep that in mind as you digest the rest of this chapter.

One of the first questions a newcomer to yoga asks is, "What should I eat?" In yoga the most important practice — after proper breathing — is proper eating. The health of the human body depends on what it is fed. A body that is fed sluggish food will be sluggish. A body that has been fed sugar and grease all its life runs a higher risk of quitting sooner than a body that has been nourished properly over the years. Most importantly, a person cannot benefit fully from the practice of yoga without first recognizing the connection between diet and health, and then doing something about it. Remember, you are what you eat.

Besides working diligently to incorporate the principles of yama and niyama into your life, and while working to perfect the breathing techniques and the asanas, you also need to adjust your eating habits to conform to the yogic lifestyle you aspire to.

The history and culture of the United States have not been conducive to the development of a healthy cuisine and conscientious eating habits. Most of us would be much better off with a few simple adjustments to the type of food we eat and our attitudes toward it.

Perhaps you have tried in the past to break an unhealthy habit—smoking, alcohol, junk food, sodas, etc.—by going "cold turkey" all on your own. You probably had some initial success, but eventually found yourself giving in to the cravings and slipping back into your old ways. This time let your study and practice of the mental and physical disciplines of yoga guide and support you in this endeavor. Practice of the yamas and niyamas will bring equilibrium to your mind and spirit, while the exercises of the asanas and pranayama will bring healing and strength to your body. You will find further support in a good yoga class in the form of friends, companions, and mentors. The most important thing is to take the first step and just do it.

> **DISCLAIMER:** *If you have a serious drug or alcohol addiction you need to seek the advice and support of a doctor, as sudden withdrawal causes serious and sometimes fatal physiological reactions. The addition of yoga to a prescribed recovery regimen will greatly enhance the outcome of the recovery plan.*

The best way to begin eating better is to substitute healthy foods and snacks for the ones you know aren't good for you. These days nearly every town in America has at least one health food store. Organic foods and healthy alternatives can be found in most supermarkets as well, either in a separate health food section or integrated among the products throughout the store. There are also many good cookbooks available covering a wide range of ingredients, techniques, and cuisines conducive to healthy eating. Contrary to what you may have heard, you do not have to be a vegan or a vegetarian to be a yogin or to be healthy, nor does healthy food exist only as expensive specialty items.

It is almost inconceivable that even though you are living in the richest, most technologically advanced country in the world, a large part of the population is starving itself to death. I'm not talking about economics; I'm talking about ignorance. The word "ignorance" comes from the root verb "to ignore." Contrary to current popular usage, an ignorant person is not one who is stupid, but is one who knows the truth and chooses to ignore it.

Almost every day, you choose to eat the wrong things, and you know you are eating the wrong things. You eat food that may taste good, but it can't be properly digested and assimilated into your body. The result is one of two things: either it passes right on through your system and out the back door taking most of its nutrients with it, or it just sits there while all of the fats, sugars, and toxins soak into the walls of your intestines and pass into your circulatory system. Your brain becomes fuzzy and your body sluggish. Your blood sugar goes up, your arteries harden, and your blood pressure rises putting a strain on your liver and kidneys, all of which lead to chronic disease and a shortened lifespan.

There Are No Quick Fixes

The natural tendency of most humans is to avoid taking personal responsibility for their lives and to look for the easy way out. When it comes to correcting the damage done by poor nutrition and lack of exercise, there is no end to diets and schemes that claim to give maximum results with minimum effort—just ask our friend, The Internet. The vast majority of the diets brought up by an internet search of "fad diets" are just plain silly, and some are potentially harmful. Most of them will work in the short term, but have no lasting effect, or will result in the dieter gaining back more weight than was lost. Many of these will also result in a reduction in your bank balance, as they often require the dieter to spend money on special foods and supplements that promise miracle results.

There are a few diets out there—for example, the South Beach, the Atkins, and the Mediterranean diets—that are nutritionally sound and result in long-term weight control and improved health. The South Beach and Atkins diets are trademarked plans with websites offering various levels of support including recipes and nutritional information for free or for a modest subscription fee.

They also make available for purchase various meal plans and other food items, but it is not difficult, is more economical, and more healthful to prepare the meals and snacks yourself.

The Mediterranean diet is not so much a diet as it is a style of eating based on the cuisine of the Mediterranean region. Many books offering background science, recipes, and practical cooking guides have been published about this diet, and there are many online articles about it as well.

The Gluten Debate

Perhaps the most controversial dietary issue to arise in recent years is the question of gluten. The number of people in this country who have a life-threatening intolerance to gluten is small. About 1% of the population has diagnosed celiac disease and 0.4% has a confirmed wheat allergy for a combined total of about two million people, and yet over three million Americans are following a gluten-free diet, with millions more conscientiously reducing their consumption of gluten. The former are people who have diagnosed themselves with what is now known as non-celiac gluten sensitivity (NCGS), while the latter are those who have become convinced that eating gluten will make them sick.

Gluten intolerance has been blamed for a broad spectrum of symptoms manifesting as a range of gastrointestinal disturbances; headaches, migraines, and "brain fog;" fatigue, fibromyalgia, and muscle and joint pain; a host of allergies and autoimmune disorders; and an array of neurological and psychiatric disorders including schizophrenia, autism, and attention deficit hyperactivity disorder. While a small portion of these people have met the criteria for a clinical diagnosis of NCGS—negative results when tested for celiac disease and wheat allergies, and improvement of symptoms after complete gluten withdrawal and the return of symptoms after gluten consumption—the majority have not. Research indicates that some of the undiagnosed who report subjective improvement on a GF diet may actually be sensitive to gluten, or they may be sensitive to some other component of the food, either another protein or a sugar that occurs naturally or one of the multitude of additives and preservatives found in processed food. Then again, the perceived improvement may be the result of a new and conscientious attention to one's eating habits; people feel better because they are making healthier food choices. It is interesting to note that the number of people following a gluten-free diet tripled between 2009 and 2016 while the number of people with celiac disease remained constant.

The gluten-free diet as we know it today is based largely on personal experience and anecdotal evidence. It has been propelled by well-funded publicity campaigns, celebrity hype and, yes, peer pressure. Every supermarket has at least one aisle lined with GF snacks, breads, and cereals, with more GF labels scattered throughout the store. Keep in mind that it is not the gluten-free food that is good for you; it's eating less food with gluten. Remember too, that gluten-free junk food is still junk food.

Some Keys to Dietary Choices

While there are no quick fixes in the area of health and health maintenance, there are some universal truths that are simple to understand and easy to put into practice, and all are a part of a perfectly balanced yogic lifestyle.

The first step toward good nutrition is to eat a variety of simple, colorful, and natural foods. Fresh ingredients purchased locally and in season are best, but not always possible. Limited or seasonal accessibility to these ideal foods, and the extra time it can take to shop for and to prepare them push us toward food that has already been processed to some degree, usually by canning or freezing.

While it is true that nutrient levels are usually highest in fresh fruits and vegetables, that only holds true if the produce is really fresh. Nutrients start to degrade as soon as the produce is harvested. Food that is destined for the cannery or the freezer is usually processed within hours of harvest, whereas fresh produce can spend three to seven days in transport and storage before it is consumed. And let's face it, how many times have you brought home that beautiful bunch of broccoli or bag of fresh green beans intending to have them for dinner that night, only to discover them two weeks later, limp and yellow in the vegetable drawer?

When selecting canned or frozen foods, be sure to read the labels. Look for ingredient lists that are short and don't include things you can't pronounce. Check to see if sugar is listed, and its position in the list. Ingredients are listed in order of their proportion by weight in the product, and the first three items make up the bulk of what you will be eating. Compare the nutritional information of your options for levels of sodium, sugar, and fats. Look for products with no added salt or sugar, but avoid those designated as "lite" as those frequently have some other artificial component added to make up for a perceived loss of flavor or texture. While fresh is best, keeping your pantry and freezer stocked with a variety of carefully selected canned, packaged, and frozen ingredients will make it easy for you to assemble tasty and wholesome meals with minimal time and effort.

What About Organic?

If you ask our friend, The Internet, you will find that the question of the nutritional superiority of organic food is open for debate. If you are making a comparison of vitamins and minerals there is essentially no difference. When it comes to antioxidants—those wonderful molecules that protect our cells, boost our immune systems, and help ward off cancer—organic comes out ahead. Another group of dietary superheroes, omega-3 fatty acids, are also found in higher concentrations in organically raised (grass fed) meat and dairy products.

Choosing organic is not just a question of nutrition. Through the miracle of modern chemistry, farmers have been equipped with an extensive arsenal of weapons to ensure that their crops will grow and that most of them will make it to market in good condition. Consequently, we unavoidably ingest a small amount of these toxins along with our food. Fortunately for us there are several government agencies working together to establish "safe" levels of these substances, and to ensure that none of them exceed these levels in our food. In this respect, the difference between conventional and organic foods is that the list of pesticides and other chemicals approved for organic farming is much shorter than the list for conventional farming. This difference is reflected in the results of studies that found fewer pesticide residues in organic foods than in conventional foods.

When it comes to bacterial contamination, one should assume that all fresh food items are a potential source. With meat and dairy products, conventional products are more likely to be a source of antibiotic-resistant strains, whereas organic products are much less likely. That difference has been attributed to the restriction of antibiotic use in animals certified for organic products, versus the regular use of antibiotics for disease prevention and growth enhancement in animals used for conventional products. With fresh produce, organic is more likely to be a source of e. coli or salmonella because of the use of manure in organic farming methods. As you can see, good hygiene is essential for the preparation of healthy food — organic or conventional; meat, dairy, or produce.

While organic produce has become more widely available in recent years, it still tends to cost more than conventionally-grown fruits and vegetables. Certain non-organic items can be nearly as safe to consume as their organic counterparts, depending on the item and its source, and it is good to know which ones when you are facing budgetary constraints or a limited selection. Consumer Reports.org presents a well-balanced discussion of this topic. To find it, go to their home page and enter "pesticides in produce" in the search bar. The article "Eat the Peach, Not the Pesticide" will be listed under "News and Articles" on the search results page. An internet search for "clean 15 and dirty dozen" will bring up links to a list of fruits and vegetables that are relatively safe as conventionally grown, and a list of those most contaminated by pesticide residues from conventional farming.

GMOs: Food Safety and Environmental Impact

The arguments on this topic range from "GMOs are perfectly safe to eat and they will prevent global starvation, and planting GMO crops will protect the environment," to "GMO crops are poison and planting them will destroy entire ecological systems." Unfortunately, there is equal evidence that can lead you to believe either of these arguments and everything in between. Part of the problem is that there is conflicting information regarding the safety of the modifications themselves. Some modifications may indeed be safe or even beneficial, such as the ones made to increase nutritional value, or the ability to grow in less hospitable conditions, but even with these there is a lack of consensus.

The most common modifications, however, involve the insertion of genetic code that will enable a plant to withstand broad and multiple applications of herbicide to kill competing weeds in the field, or the insertion of a gene to make a toxin that will kill insect pests that eat the crop, or both. In these cases, the issue is far more complex than simply the health and safety of the consumer; these modifications introduce potentially critical challenges not just to our health, but to the environment, agricultural economics, and cultures worldwide as well.

The yogic principle of ahimsa asks that you do no harm. Your decision to avoid genetically modified foods and to choose foods produced by following sustainable and humane organic methods will strengthen the foundation of your life as a yogin.

How Do I Know What I Am Eating?

As of the publication of this book, sixty-four countries including most of the European Union, Japan, Australia, Brazil, Russia, and China require labeling of genetically modified food. The United States, Canada, and Mexico do not. What we do have in the United States are two labels that alert us to products that contain verifiably minimal amounts of modified DNA. Products bearing the USDA Organic label have been certified as having been produced according to approved methods and as meeting specific standards as verified by a USDA-accredited agent. One of these standards is that GMOs are prohibited in organic products. This means that organic grains and produce cannot originate with GMO seeds, animals used for the production of organic meat and dairy cannot eat feed made from GMO alfalfa, corn or soy, and processed food cannot contain any GMO ingredients — and that's in addition to all the other requirements for organic certification. The other label that can guide you to foods and other products that meet their standards is granted by the Non-GMO Project, a not-for-profit organization dedicated to creating a standardized definition for non-GMO products in the North American food industry. This label verifies only that the product meets the Projects standards for levels of modified DNA. In other words, all products labeled USDA Organic are non-GMO, but products labeled Non-GMO are not necessarily organic unless also labeled as such.

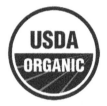 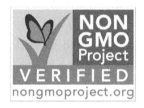

What Should I Eat?

The USDA has been issuing information on food and nutrition since 1894. Initially, the information was published in pamphlet or booklet form. 1943 saw the introduction of the first in a series of attempts to present guidelines for dietary choices as illustrative pie charts, block diagrams and pyramids of various complexity and, at times, questionable nutritional guidance.

The current iteration—MyPlate—is not perfect but it is a good place to start. The image encourages you to visualize your daily intake laid out as portions on a plate. Ideally, half of your plate should contain servings of vegetables and fruits, with more veggies than fruit; the other half should be grains and proteins, heavy on the grain relative to the protein. Dairy is served on the side, and the image has no reference to fats and oils at all.

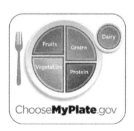

The first thing you need to do is to stop thinking of a healthy diet in terms of what you shouldn't eat—think instead of things you should eat. By focusing on a balanced assortment of healthy foods, you won't have room for the unhealthy ones.

Imagine *YourPlate* not as a two-dimensional graphic composed of flat, featureless blocks, but as a richly-hued work of art painted with details evoking multiple textures and suggestive of a variety of flavors and aromas. Just as an artist paints a picture with pigments of red, yellow, and blue, blending them and "seasoning" them with black and white, we will paint our plate with vegetables, fruits, grains, and proteins, and will use dairy and healthy fats and oils to blend, stretch, and highlight the picture.

There are many good resources available on line and in print that provide detailed information about the foods that comprise the various groups, including their nutritional value and guides for selection and preparation.

Details about each food group—what's in it, recommended daily servings, serving sizes, etc.—can be found at ChooseMyPlate. gov. Note: enter the address in the address bar of your web browser rather than the search bar, otherwise it can be difficult to find. Links to each of the food groups can be found by hovering over the first item—"MYPLATE"—in the main menu on the home page. The information is basic, but it is useful in helping you to form a visual image of the food you eat, and an organized way of thinking about your diet.

Out of the multitude of websites dedicated to healthy eating, one stands out as a source of useful and reliable information: The World's Healthiest Foods (whfoods.org). This site provides an in-depth discussion of each of the "100 World's Healthiest Foods," a list that spans all of the food groups, and includes a selection of herbs and spices as well. The information regarding health benefits and nutritional value is quite detailed and is drawn from published peer-reviewed scientific research. Each listing also includes practical information on selection and storage, preparation and cooking, and menu suggestions and recipes. This site also has an extensive and growing list of articles covering a range of topics relevant to healthy eating.

Vegetables: Cooked or Raw?

While there is no argument that vegetables are good for you, there is some disagreement as to whether they are healthier cooked or raw. The answer is yes, they are. Some nutrients and enzymes are destroyed by the heat of cooking, while others are made more available by the process. Cooking also develops flavors, aromas, and textures different from those of the raw foods. A healthy and appealing diet will contain a mixture of both cooked and raw foods.

A few tips on preparation:

- Let the vegetables sit for five to ten minutes before cooking or serving raw. The act of cutting releases some nutrients and enzymes that can aid digestion.
- Use as little water as possible. Cook by steaming, or by "sautéing" in a small amount of water or broth; a little olive oil can be added at the end before serving.
- Cook vegetables until tender, but not soft. Watch the color develop as they cook; nutrition is at its peak when the color is most vivid.

Potatoes: Not Just Empty Calories

While potatoes are often one of the first things to be ditched when one resolves to eat healthier, that is actually not a good idea. What you do want to leave behind are greasy French fries and chips, sour cream, butter, and cheese toppings, and rich cream gravies. The potato itself—steamed, baked, or roasted—is an excellent source of vitamins, minerals, and fiber, especially if the skin is included. It also provides a respectable amount of complete protein—a rare thing in the vegetable world. A wholesome and satisfying meal can be quickly composed with a baked or steamed potato, some steamed broccoli, and a dollop of Greek yogurt; add a drizzle of olive oil and a sprinkling of feta cheese for a little more flavor.

Whole Grains

You all know by now that whole grains are not just better for you than refined grains, they are really good for you; a quick search of the internet will lead you to numerous well-supported discussions of that fact. Briefly, whole grains deliver more nutrients including fiber, protein, vitamins—especially B vitamins—and minerals. Replacing refined grains in your diet with whole grains can help to regulate your blood pressure, reduce your risk of type 2 diabetes, and improve your digestion.

That said, there are times when the aesthetics of a meal are best when accompanied by white rice, or crusty white bread. The occasional indulgence will not hurt you, and can facilitate the consumption and enhance the enjoyment of a carefully prepared composition of nutritious food.

Protein

Proteins are large, complex molecules that are required for the structure, function, and regulation of all living things. These infinitely diverse functional units are all constructed from just twenty small components called amino acids. While our own bodies can produce most of the amino acids, we need to consume proteins in our food in order to supply sufficient amino acids for the growth, repair, and regulation of our bodies. In addition, there are several amino acids required by us that are only available from dietary sources. The protein foods page of ChooseMyPlate.gov is a good place to start looking for basic information such as how much protein is needed daily, and how much protein is in various amounts of different kinds of food, including non-vegetarian, vegetarian, and vegan sources.

Meat and Poultry:

If you choose to eat meat, do so sparingly. Look for grass-fed beef, and free-range poultry; these choices are not only a more healthful product, but they have been raised following more humane practices. If you live in an area where you can buy directly from the farmer, then so much the better.

Fish

Fish is one of the healthiest things you can eat—just ask our friend, The Internet—but some fish are better choices than others. It is well known that certain types of fish accumulate significant levels of toxic substances in their bodies—not just mercury, but antibiotics and other chemical pollutants as well. Also, the populations of some varieties of fish are declining as a result of overfishing, pollution, and other ecological pressures. For help in making healthy and ecologically sound seafood choice, check out the Monterey Bay Aquarium Seafood Watch at seafoodwatch.org, and the Environmental Defense Fund Seafood Selector at seafood.edf.org.

Legumes: Beans, Peas, and Lentils

This vegetable group presents a substantial amount of protein in a variety of colors, sizes, and shapes, which makes them a good foundation for vegetarian meals. They are, however, lacking in one or more of the essential amino acids. If your diet includes meat, dairy or seafood on a regular basis, that won't be a problem. If you are following a vegetarian or vegan diet, you will need to include another plant protein such as nuts, or whole grains that will fill in the missing pieces.

To Soy, or Not To Soy?

There are numerous articles written by the internet wellness gurus that warn against the consumption of soy beans in any form—with the possible exception of the fermented products, tempeh, miso, and natto—describing a range of ill effects. The truth is that there are many studies reporting conflicting results, with the most recent data seeming to show a positive effect or none at all. This would suggest that the inclusion of whole soy products as part of a balanced diet is of overall benefit. A detailed and technical review of the topic can be found at the Linus Pauling Institute, Micronutrient Information Center (lpi.oregonstate.edu/mic). From the menu on the home page, select "Articles" > "Dietary Factors" > "Phytochemicals" > "Soy Isoflavones." For a good explanation in layman's terms, and some tips on what to look for when choosing—or avoiding—soy products, put "Dr. Oz Soy" into a Google search; that will bring up links to three short videos and an article that address the issues in a balanced and intelligent manner.

The main things to be aware of when choosing soy products are:
- Look for certified organic, non-GMO
- Choose whole or minimally processed soy.
- Avoid products with ingredients listed as soy protein, soy protein isolate, fractionated soy protein, soy isoflavone, or any combination of those words.

Dairy

Dairy products are a valuable source of nutrients including protein, minerals—especially calcium and phosphorus—an array of B-complex vitamins, and vitamins A, D, E, and K. The easiest way to include dairy in your diet is to have a glass of milk. If you are lactose intolerant, try regular or Greek-style plain yogurt or dairy kefir; you will be getting all of the benefits of a glass of milk, plus a healthy dose of probiotic bacteria. Be sure to look for brands containing live cultures. Also, avoid flavored yogurts as they can carry a heavy load of sugar or artificial sweeteners. It is quite easy and much healthier to add honey, fruit, and other flavors to your own taste.

If you are considering non-fat dairy because you think it is healthier, think again. Unless you have a compelling reason to avoid fats, full fat or 2% is a better choice, particularly if the product is from grass-fed cows. The amount of fat added to a well balanced diet is not that much. In addition, many of the most beneficial nutrients in milk are fat-soluble and are most abundant and available in full-fat or 2% fat products. Another benefit of full-fat dairy is that it will keep you feeling satisfied longer than the non-fat version, cutting down on the urge to snack later. Again, as with meat, always look for organic and choose grass-fed whenever possible. Dairy products produced with these standards are not only more healthful, but confer more humane treatment to the animals as well.

Fats and Oils (Lipids):

Fats are a necessary component of a healthy diet. They are required for proper brain function and nerve health, as well as normal growth and development. They are also the key structural component of the cellular membrane. One fat in particular, cholesterol, is the precursor of a host of hormones that regulate metabolism, growth, and reproduction. Some essential nutrients are fat-soluble — that is, they are found in the fats and oils of the food we eat, and require the presence of fat in order to be properly absorbed by our bodies. In addition, much of the flavor and satisfaction we find in our food is derived from the fat it contains.

While much of the food we eat naturally contains fats and/or oils, we often add more during the preparation, and that's what gets us in trouble. A full discussion of what fat is and what fats we should and shouldn't be eating is beyond the scope of this chapter. To learn more, put "What is fat?" and "What are good fats?" into a Google search. I highly recommend an article found on WebMD, "The Skinny on Fat: Good Fats vs. Bad Fats," (webmd.com/diet/obesity/features/skinny-fat-good-fats-bad-fats#4), and a series of articles found on the Verywell website beginning with "Dietary Fat: Definitions and Examples" (verywell.com/what-is-dietary-fat-3496105).

When it comes to choosing an oil for cooking, you can't go wrong with extra virgin olive oil (EVOO). A number of the internet wellness gurus will try to tell you that if you cook with EVOO it will cause toxins to form that will ultimately cause cancer or make you ill. That is not true; at worst it may reduce the level of some of the components that make olive oil especially healthful. The composition of olive oil is such that it holds up well under most cooking conditions; it even works well in most baked goods. The World's Healthiest Foods website has a complete and well-supported discussion of this; look for "Olive Oil" in the sidebar menu of the homepage. If the recipe requires an oil with a more delicate flavor, canola oil is a good choice. Look for organic, expeller-pressed or cold-pressed to avoid GMOs and certain toxins found in non-organic extraction processes. Canola oil is also good for cooking with high heat, such as in a wok or high-heat roasting. For the occasional recipe that requires a solid fat such as for a flaky pie crust or biscuits, use palm oil. Be sure to choose one that is certified by the Roundtable on Sustainable Palm Oil (rspo.org).

We Are Not Alone: Probiotics and Prebiotics

Our guts are populated by a vast and varied assortment of bacteria — up to four and a half pounds worth. They don't just live there, they have a relationship that is mutually beneficial to them and to us — we give them a cozy place to live and food to eat, and they help keep us healthy. The microbiome, as this population is called, benefits us in a number of ways: it generates substances that aid digestion; it inhibits the overgrowth of "bad" organisms that can make us ill; it synthesizes vitamins such as vitamin K and the B vitamins, folate, B-12, and biotin. It also helps to breakdown and remove carcinogens found in our food — and that's just for starters. The influence of the microbiome extends beyond the gut, affecting our body's glucose production and storage, immune system, and possibly even our mood and state of mind.

Probiotics are bacteria that, when consumed, add to and support the "good" bacteria in your gut. Prebiotics are the fiber compounds that pass through your stomach and small intestine undigested and become food for the microbiome in your large intestine. These prebiotics and probiotics can be found packaged up in convenient — and expensive — capsules, powders, and liquids, that occupy yards of prime shelf space at the health food store. If you are in relative good health and are eating according to the principles laid out in · this chapter, these supplements are unnecessary. The vegetables and fruits, whole grains, and legumes serve up a healthy portion of prebiotics to keep your microbiome well fed. Yogurt, kefir, and cheeses such as Cheddar, Swiss, Gouda, and Parmesan, as well as sauerkraut and other fermented foods are prepared with bacteria that will help to keep your internal population of bacteria on the "good" side. These foods contain live cultures and will be found in the refrigerated section of grocery stores. Yogurt, kefir, and fermented vegetables such as sauerkraut and pickles are not hard to make yourself — there are numerous guides and recipes to be found in books and on the internet—and their preparation is a good way to develop greater awareness and control over the food you eat.

A Note About Supplements

As with probiotics and prebiotics, if you are eating according to the guidelines of this chapter, you will be better off spending your money on better food than on dietary supplements. Most of the vitamins, minerals, and other nutritional factors require the presence of other factors to work properly, or even to work at all. Consuming more than necessary is at least a waste of money, as your body will simply dump what it does not need. Some vitamins can cause serious health problems if taken in excess, and some can interfere with medications you may be taking. An excellent article on this topic—"Know the Difference Between Fat- and Water-Soluble Nutrients"—can be found on the WebMD website (webmd.com/vitamins-and-supplements/nutrition-vitamins-11/ fat-water-nutrient).

Rules To Eat By

How you eat is as important as what you eat. By following these recommended practices you will derive the maximum benefits from the food you eat. You will experience not only better digestion and utilization of nutrients, but increased enjoyment of your food and pleasure at mealtime, all of which lead to better health and well-being for your body, mind, and soul.

Eat slowly

By taking smaller bites and chewing them thoroughly before swallowing, you will not only be better preparing the food for digestion, but you will also be able to truly savor the aromas, flavors, and textures—to really enjoy and appreciate your food.

It takes about twenty minutes for the stomach to signal to the brain that food is moving through the system. There is a complex cross talk of neurotransmitters and hormones that develops during the course of a meal to prepare the digestive system for the arrival of food, activate various metabolic pathways, and stimulate feelings of satisfaction and pleasure after eating. If we eat too fast this system is bypassed and we wind up feeling full and bloated rather than contented and nourished.

The benefits of eating slowly are many, including:

1. **Appetite reduction and portion size control**
   Your appetite will be sated long before you have eaten everything in sight, and by savoring every bite, you will derive more pleasure from smaller portions.

2. **Weight reduction**
   The logical result of point 1 is that you will gain control of your weight.

3. **Better food**
   When you eat slow enough to savor your food and think about what you are eating, you will begin to make better food choices.

4. **Better digestion**
   The first step in digestion is chewing. Chewing mechanically breaks food into small pieces and mixes it with saliva. Enzymes in saliva begin the chemical process of digestion. Thorough chewing makes the subsequent steps of digestion easier and more efficient, which leads to the next point:

5. **Reduction of heartburn and gastroesophageal reflux**
   Eating too fast can contribute to acid reflux. Thorough chewing and careful swallowing — slower eating — can help to control this issue.

6. **Better management of blood sugar levels**
   A meal eaten slowly will raise your blood sugar levels less than the same meal eaten quickly. Carbohydrates begin to be broken down into sugar almost as soon as you put them in your mouth, and these sugars enter the bloodstream quickly. Eating slowly will help to keep your body's sugar processing capacity from being overwhelmed, and will allow time to mobilize the insulin and receptors needed to move the sugars out of circulation and into your cells to be converted to energy.

7. **You will make the cook happy**

It takes an effort of inspiration, planning, acquisition, preparation, and service to prepare a meal—from the simplest pot of soup to the most elaborate banquet. Nothing makes a cook happier than to see faces reflecting pleasure derived from the food that has been lovingly prepared and presented. A happy cook is a good cook; express your pleasure by lingering over each bite. If you are cooking for yourself, relax and take the time to enjoy the fruits of your labor; it will make you a better cook (see point 3).

Reflect on the source of your meal and ask God to bless it

All food is a gift from God, regardless of Who or What you imagine God to be. In addition, all food was once alive (e.g. meat and vegetables) or was taken from living entities (e.g. milk, honey, and eggs). As you are giving thanks to God for your food and asking for His blessing on it, consider the living beings from which it is derived and give thanks for the sacrifices made for the sake of your nourishment. You can never ask God for too many blessings, and you can never thank God too much; that is a universal Truth.

Taking the time at the start of each meal to express your gratitude will give your body, mind, and spirit an opportunity to step away from the demands of the world and leave behind your anxieties over the things you lack. Focus instead on the sufficiency before you. This simple ritual is an effective way to activate the yama of aparigraha—don't be greedy—in your life and in the lives of your whole family. Greed becomes gluttony when referring to food, and food consumed with that motivation might as well be poison, whereas each bite of food tasted and savored with an attitude of thanksgiving will give to you every bit of goodness it contains.

Do not overeat

Just as aparigraha is demonstrated by the practice of giving thanks at the start of a meal, brahmacharya—don't waste energy—is exhibited when one heeds the caution to refrain from overeating.

Overeating is, indeed, a waste of energy on several levels. It takes energy to grow, process, and transport the food that will become a meal. Then more energy is used to acquire the ingredients, assemble, cook, and serve them, and to clean up afterward.

Our bodies expend energy just by maintaining the basic functions of life such as breathing, thinking, circulation, digestion, etc. Think of it like an engine that is turned on and idling without going anywhere; it still uses gas. When we are active—going somewhere—we need more energy, just as your car uses more gas when it is moving down the highway. Whether your car is sitting in the driveway with its engine idling or being driven across the country, it will run out of gas (energy) sooner or later and you will fill it up again. Similarly, your body needs to be refueled whether you have been sitting still reading a book or out running a marathon. The big difference between you and your car in this respect is that your car has a fuel tank that will only hold a certain amount and no more. If you try to put more into the tank, most fuel pumps will automatically shut off to prevent the gasoline from spilling out onto the ground. Your car cannot "eat" more fuel than it needs.

On the other hand, we are capable of ingesting far more fuel than our energy expenditure requires. When we do that, the extra is converted to a form that is easily stored until we need it to support an increase in activity—it becomes fat. Throughout our history, and to this day in many places around the world, the ability to store fuel acquired in a time of plenty has made the difference between life and death when sufficient food is not available. For those of us living in this time and place of relative abundance and lack of physical challenge, these stores of potential energy (fat) are seldom dipped into and tend to accumulate. The result is the increasing incidence of cardiovascular disease, stroke, diabetes and other metabolic disorders. This marvelous strategy for survival has become a threat to our health and well-being.

Over eating is wasteful of energy and resources on a non-personal level—that is on a global, community, and family level—while on a personal level it is wasteful of our vitality and good health. By exercising the principles of brahmacharya—don't waste your energy; practice self-control—you can reverse the trend.

Avoid eating heavily before going to bed

The process of digestion is most efficient when your body is in an upright position — sitting, standing, walking, etc.— and it takes about three hours for your food to make its way out of your stomach and into your intestines. Reclining for sleep while your stomach is full slows down that progress and can cause or aggravate acid reflux and other feelings of discomfort or even sleep apnea. As a result, you can't sleep, or if you can, your sleep is disrupted and unrestful. There are even reports that link reclining or going to sleep following a heavy meal with an increased risk of stroke.

You need seven to nine hours of quality sleep each night for the restoration of your body and mind. Loss of sleep affects your memory, your coordination, and the ability to focus your attention and to control your emotions. It also has serious consequences for your immune and endocrine systems, and contributes to obesity, diabetes, and hypertension.

The best solution is to make lunch the main meal of your day and keep dinner as light as possible, finishing no less than three hours before bedtime. If you are someone who wakes up hungry in the middle of the night, try having a small snack about thirty minutes before going to bed. Whole grain cereal with milk is an excellent choice, and the internet has more good suggestions; do a search for "food to eat before going to bed." Just remember to keep it small — under 100 or 200 calories.

Don't allow negative energies to intrude into your mealtime.

The process of eating involves more than just putting food in your mouth, chewing, and swallowing; it is a complex activity that requires your full attention if you are to gain the maximum benefit from it. As discussed in the first rule, eat slowly, your physiological responses to food take time and considerable cross-talk between your body and your mind to gear up into full digestion mode. When your mind is subjected to outside distractions such as TV, texting, etc., that line of communication is broken. Your focus is shifted away from the enjoyment of the flavors, textures, and aromas of the food, and you loose the link that carries the signals of fullness and satisfaction between your stomach and your brain. That kind of thoughtless consumption leads to eating too much and to inefficient digestion.

Besides just being a mental distraction, watching television can divert your body's energy away from the process of digestion. A portion of your nervous system is dedicated to the regulation and control of your internal organs and bodily functions. When you are relaxed, blood flow to the gastrointestinal tract is increased, gastric fluids are secreted, the wavelike constriction of the intestines (peristalsis) is stimulated, your mouth is moist with saliva, your breathing and heartbeat is slow and steady, and your muscles are relaxed—all conditions that promote digestion.

When you turn on the TV, you are immediately assaulted by a flow of negative energy and destructive frequencies. You become mentally involved in whatever is being broadcast—the news, a sporting competition, a thrilling adventure, heart-stopping action, or gut-wrenching drama. Even though you are watching from the security of your own home, and even though you know that what you are seeing is only a game or just a story, your brain is telling your body to gear up for a physical challenge. Your breathing, heart rate, and blood pressure increase; production of saliva and gastric fluids is reduced; peristalsis slows and your muscles tense. Your brain reroutes the resources of your body toward those systems and functions that are necessary for survival and—in the short term—digestion isn't one of them. Eating should be a time of peace and rest so that the digestive process can kick in and do the job it was intended to do.

These physiological responses occur whether the distraction is television, loud or aggressive music, or squabbles around the dinner table, and their impact on your health is cumulative—the longer you continue these behaviors, the more your body, mind, and spirit suffer the consequences. Exposure to the destructive energy frequencies that permeate the world today—various entertainments, sports, current events, hatred and anger, random noise—cannot be avoided all together, but the effect on you can be alleviated by putting into practice the principles of yoga as outlined in previous chapters.

Your home can become a haven of tranquility and mealtime can become a ritual that taps into the universal creative frequency, bringing peace to your spirit and health to your body.

Don't drink cold liquids with your meals.

Ingesting large quantities of cold liquid during the course of a meal runs the risk of interfering with the digestive process. On the other hand, drinking a glass of room temperature or warm liquid about a half an hour before or after — or both — can have a beneficial effect on digestion.

Digestion takes place best at the temperature found in your stomach, and on food that has been thoroughly chewed and carefully swallowed. Liquids are often used during the course of a meal to wash down mouthfuls of food that have been improperly chewed and are not ready to be introduced to the stomach — see Eat Slowly, point 4. Pausing during a meal to take a sip or two of tepid water or other liquid is a good way to slow down the pace of a meal. If you find yourself needing larger quantities of water to swallow your food, slow down and take smaller bites. It is also possible that you may be mildly dehydrated and need to increase your fluid intake during the course of the day.

Allow at least 5-10 minutes to pass after eating before resuming activities.

While there are no hard and fast rules concerning how long you should wait after a meal before resuming your activities or engaging in exercise, it is wise to rest at the table for a few minutes after eating.

Remember from the discussion warning against negative energies while eating that digestion takes place most efficiently while the body is relaxed and at rest. Too much activity too soon can pull your body's resources away from digestion and slow it down. Take a few minutes at the end of your meal to allow your food to settle and to begin to move smoothly through the process. As you return to a state of activity, do so gradually to allow your body to make a smooth transition from relaxation to action.

While this practice has obvious physiological benefits, it conveys spiritual benefits as well. When dining with others, it can be a time of congenial conversation. Lingering around the table is also a compliment to the cook. If you are dining alone, it is an excellent time for meditation on the blessings in your life. Cleaning up or assisting with the clean up after a meal is not only an opportunity to practice karma yoga, but is also an excellent way to help your body make the transition from a sedentary state to an active one.

Share your food with those who have little.

It is the practice of karma yoga that elevates the yogic path above the level of a simple regimen for self-improvement. The central tenet of karma yoga is to serve or give to others not with the chance of a reward for one's self, but because it is the right thing to do. This idea that is found in the teachings of most of the religions in this world is neatly summarized in what we know of as the Golden Rule:

> *So in everything, do unto others what you would have them do to you, for this sums up the Law and the Prophets. Matthew 7:12 (NIV)*

What service can be of greater value than to provide nourishment to others by sharing with them from your abundance?

How about your neighbors? Does the little old lady at the end of the street have family or friends that visit regularly? Are the children of the single mother next door getting enough to eat? Why not "adopt" them and help to meet their needs until they can take care of themselves.

If you don't personally know of anyone in need there are churches and other charitable organizations based in your community that can either connect you with a person or family, or will welcome your gift of money, food, or service in aid of their mission. You need to do a little homework to find an organization or program that reliably and efficiently does what it says it will do, and whose mission is one that you can fully support. Look around your own community first; ask people like your child's teacher or school administrator, a local radio or television station, your pastor or other church leaders will likely have first hand knowledge of people in need and the charities that can help. Search the internet for more broadly-based organizations on the national and international level. In general, faith-based benevolence organizations such as Samaritan's Purse, Catholic Charities, and the Salvation Army—to name just a few—tend to have a good history of effective disbursement of their funds. There are several websites—Charity Navigator, Charity Watch, Give.org, or GuideStar—where you can find ratings and information on thousands of charitable organizations.

When considering sharing your food, don't forget the animals that live among us as companions, helpers, and friends. Monetary gifts to local animal rescue facilities and organizations are always welcome, but sometimes gifts of food, bedding, litter, and other supplies are needed; check with your local shelter to see what is appropriate. You might also consider working with a local rescue organization as a foster family for pets that are difficult to place, such as an aged dog or cat that needs a loving home to live out its final days, a pair that are closely bonded and would suffer if separated, one that needs to recover from illness or injury, or one that needs to be rehabilitated from an abusive situation. It might also be that your elderly neighbor living on a shoestring is not comfortable accepting charity for his or her own needs, but would be grateful for gifts of food and treats, grooming, or even a trip to the veterinarian for his or her beloved companion.

Regardless of what you have to give, or to whom you choose to give it, the fundamental spirit of this rule is to GIVE. Period. Give on a regular basis, and give without question. It will be a blessing not only to those who receive, but to you as well, for having made the sacrifice to help another in need.

Know Where Your Food Comes From

Read the labels on packaged foods. Ask questions of the produce manager and the butcher at your favorite store. Talk to the vendors at the farmers' market. The more you know about your food, the more wisely you can make choices based on health, nutrition, ethics, and sustainability. Try to purchase products locally and in season. There are several websites that can help you find markets, farmers, co-ops, etc. in your area. These two seem to be the most useful and user friendly: Local Harvest (localharvest.org), and Eat Well Guide (eatwellguide.org).

Of course, the best way to develop a relationship with your food is to produce it yourself. You can grow a pot of herbs on your windowsill, or plant tomatoes in a pot on the balcony. Raised beds are a good way to get maximum use from a small space. If you have a bit more room, you might even consider raising a few chickens or even a beehive. If farming is not your thing, try making your own yogurt, kefir, or sourdough. The possibilities of fermented vegetables go way beyond simple pickles and sauerkraut. Even if you try these things for a short while or just as an experiment, you will be strengthening your connection with the creative and life-sustaining frequencies.

6

Silence, Meditation, and Prayer

Years ago I conducted a simple experiment. I placed a lawn chair in the middle of my beautiful back garden, sat down, and did nothing but sit and listen for silence; for the sound of nothing.

I sat under my huge old English Walnut Tree and paid close attention to all the sounds heard on any summer afternoon in the back garden of any home located at the edge of any moderate-sized town in Southern California. I kept a careful record of the sounds I heard and of the moments of silence between sounds, noting whether the sounds were manufactured — noise — or natural. Most animal sounds such as bird-song, rustling leaves, and insects were noted as non-intrusive and therefore not noise. Dogs barking, however, I classified as noise, since noisy dogs are, largely, an artifact of human habitation. There are pets in every neighborhood whose owners have left them alone all day while they are at work. The poor dogs are lonely and bored, and have nothing better to do than to yap at every butterfly that floats by.

The results of this experiment were disturbing. I sat for over three hours, and I was not able to note a single moment without noise during that time. Not ONE! Every second of every minute was punctuated by the sound of a car going by, a siren, a truck engine idling, the honk of a horn, an airplane flying over, the bark of several dogs, children yelling at each other, phones ringing through open windows, voices, TVs and radios turned up loud, lawn mowers — anything and everything but silence.

I didn't expect much — it was Southern California, after all — but I wasn't prepared for the complete lack of silence. And this wasn't a weekend or a holiday or the evening rush hour; it was a typical mid-week afternoon when most people are at work or school.

Where can we go, if not to our own homes, to immerse ourselves in the silence of God? Shouldn't every human being be allowed a few moments of total silence per day at the very least?

Most people today have never really experienced silence, and seem almost to actively avoid it by filling the relative quiet of their moments of solitude with the sound of the computer, TV or radio. On the way to work, the noise of the road is overlaid with loud music from the car stereo. Some people seem to fear the possibility of silence so much that they carry their favorite noise with them and plug it directly into their ears everywhere they go.

We have also allowed certain sounds to invade our lives and take control. These intrusive sounds penetrate the buzz of the background and punctuate our personal soundtracks. Sounds like alarm clocks, cell phone ring tones, and announcements from computers and smart phones proclaiming the arrival of emails and text messages have attained status as immediate demands on our time and attention, regardless of any other activity we may be engaged in at the moment.

Over the past seventy years our children have been conditioned to ever increasing noise and distraction. The popularity of entertainments in the form of television programing, movies, and sporting events seems to be in direct proportion to the level of noise, action, and violence on display. Children have easy access to all of this at home through televisions, computers, and personal electronic devices, often without parental supervision or guidance.

Outside the home, at the market or the shopping mall, more machines, more chatter, other people's rude children, angry adults, rattling shopping carts, and really bad piped-in music assault our ears. It seems that our culture has developed a compulsion to fill every available space with some kind of constructed noise designed to distract us and to manipulate our mood and behavior. Even parking lots now have loud piped in music to serenade your car while you are in the store. How silly is that?

It's not just that noise is ubiquitous, but much of it is excessively loud. The last time I went to the movie theater—something I rarely do—I saw a science fiction movie with lots of action and, unbelievably, almost no violence or explosions. Even so, the sound track was so loud I had to put cotton in my ears to able to understand much of the dialogue. It is simply unnecessary. And how about the off the scale sound level at a rock concert or at the local bar?

In short, humans are accosted by more noise than they should have to bear, and they are doing it to themselves on purpose. It is no wonder the number of hearing impaired among the human species is rising.

The link between noise and stress-related disease is undeniable; just do an internet search for "noise and stress". Numerous studies have shown that a constant battering of noise causes an increase in the production of stress-related hormones. Given time, this can lead to high blood pressure and all of its consequences. Even if you get used to a high level of noise, the adaptations your body has to make are still occurring and can have a negative effect on your endocrine, immune, and cardiovascular systems.

The impact of noise pollution goes beyond physiological effects. Sleep disturbance, fatigue, irritability, aggression, annoyance and aggravation can lead to breakdowns in the bonds between family members, the development of violent behavior, and even increased criminal activity. The inability to concentrate in a noisy environment results in poor job performance. Children subjected to higher levels of noise at home and at school lag in cognitive development and spoken communication. The list of consequences is nearly endless.

It seems then, that silence is absolutely necessary for one's well-being. You cannot live, let alone live well, without it. Yet, how are you to obtain it? Where do you look? If you cannot experience it within the sanctity of your own home and garden, where can it be found?

The only solution is to look within. If silence cannot be achieved in your physical world, it must be sought on some other plane of existence. The Apostle Paul tells us in 1 Corinthians 6:19, *"Your body is the Temple of the Holy Spirit,"* and that we are to treat it with respect and not defile it with immoral acts. The same words of Truth apply here as well. The dictionary defines "temple" as "a place devoted to a special or exalted purpose," — a *place*, not necessarily a building. The innermost part of the temple is a place of peace and quiet, where one can find solitude and safety from the world — a sanctuary. You can learn to create that sanctuary within the temple of your body.

It is within the abilities of all of us to attain the highest goal of becoming a temple for Creator's Will. It requires commitment to the path, and patience along the way. The ability to create for ourselves moments of dedicated silence throughout the day is central to this achievement. Even the busiest of days contains many "in-between" moments: between phone calls, between conversations, between tasks and appointments, between destinations, etc. Each of these moments is an opportunity to enter your personal temple and take refuge in the silence of your personal sanctuary.

There are tens of thousands of constructions serving as temples scattered around the globe. There are the modern temples dedicated to acquisition and popular culture that we know as shopping malls, movie theaters, and sporting venues. They are filled with crowds, noise, chaos, greed, and often violence. These days, many places of worship have come to fall into this category, offering rock bands during services and even Starbucks and McDonald's in the lobby.

Then there are the TRUE temples; the great cathedrals, the old stone churches, the standing stones, and stone circles. Add to these the most genuine of temples; places like the old-growth groves of the Smokey Mountains, the magnificent redwood groves of the Pacific Coast, the hidden palm oases of the deserts—you get the picture. These are all places where one is naturally moved to proceed with silence and awe. What kind of temple have you built for yourself?

The point is, you can't behave like monks and nuns all day, but you do carry a temple within you. It is up to you to build and maintain the solemn and sacred atmosphere of that sanctuary, and to set aside a few moments each day to seek refuge within the temple of your own spirit—within your body-mind—in order to experience the healing peace and silence that can be found there.

You must take the time to seek silence for yourself. It can be a matter of life or death, both physically and spiritually. Anyone can communicate with God under any circumstance and in any situation, but it is good to be alone with God once in a while in order to purify your soul which is being bombarded every moment of every day with worldly nonsense—the graffiti of the human mind.

So, how do you do it? How can you produce such an environment inside your mind? It isn't that difficult, but it is even easier
if you can create a physical space where you can take your body,
where your soul and mind will be able to find the solitude and
silence necessary to be alone with God.

Your Sacred Spot

Set apart a place in your home where a level of relative silence
and solitude can be established. It doesn't need to be very big; a
small room, or part of one that can be cleared of clutter, an empty
closet, any place in the house where you can separate yourself from
the material world that commands most of your time and provides
most of your mental graffiti. You only need a small space where you
can hide away for as long as you are able, in which you can escape
from your busy schedule.

Regardless of its size or location, there is only one require-
ment for your sacred spot. Be it a closet, the attic, or the corner of
a bedroom, it must remain pure, because in this place you will be
devoting yourself to special and exalted purposes. Here you will be
talking alone, with God.

By pure, I mean simple. Your sacred spot should be stripped
bare of ALL worldly items. Even if you simply screen off the corner
of your bedroom, that corner must remain devoid of any reminder
of the outside world. There must be no competition between God
and technology. No telephones, smart phones, magazines, electronic devices, shoes, pens and papers, lamps — nothing. It doesn't
matter if the rest of your house is a mess, your sacred spot should
be a sanctuary of order, simplicity, and peace. It should be the one
place where you, and *only* you are allowed to enter, in order to
communicate with God. Got it?

Your sacred spot should be holier than any church you have
ever been in. It belongs to you and to God alone. It does not belong
to the religion or denomination you grew up in. It does not belong
to the latest New Age fad. It does not belong to any worldly philosophy. It does not belong to your friends or your family. It belongs
to you and God, and to no one else.

It should contain nothing that relates to, or even suggests any worldly faith, philosophy or religion. No religious magazines or books, no pictures of saints or any human beings that have been given "holy" status. Not even a Bible, or holy book of any religion. *Nothing* produced on this world should be allowed inside your sacred spot. Just you and God: a bare ceiling, a bare floor, four bare walls—you and God.

Silence has a function even more important than relieving stress or inducing peace of mind. It is a key factor to the attainment of your spiritual awakening. I use the term "awakening" rather than "enlightenment" because one must first wake up to the fact that one is already enlightened. Awakening to the realization of personal enlightenment is one of the first steps on the path to a yogic lifestyle. Don't let anyone try to convince you that you need to pay large sums of money, join cultic groups, or take courses to "receive enlightenment". Enlightenment is within you and all you have to do is accept that fact and move on with your life. The yogic lifestyle presented in this book is simple to follow and can be modified to meet the needs of anyone reading it. In reality, the mere fact that you are reading this book shows that you have already entered into your own awareness of personal enlightenment, and you are determined now to go forward in order to better your own spiritual and physical health and well-being.

Silence is essential for effective meditation, contemplation, or prayer—which are all basically the same thing. Your mind must be free from timetables, checklists, unresolved arguments, bad memories, politics, attitudes and opinions. Do your best to insulate your sacred spot from outside sounds, and don't even think about bringing any sounds in with you. When you enter your sacred spot for the purpose of meditation, turn off your cell phone and leave your iPods and mp3 players in another room. You have created this space and this time for a private and focused opportunity to be alone with God. When you bring music in with you, you are no longer alone; you have brought a crowd of strangers into your most private place. At best, the music is a distraction from what should be the central point of your contemplation. Worse than that, however, is the likelihood that the music will carry with it conflicting, materialistic, and negative energies from the people who wrote, performed, and produced it. You have chosen your sacred spot carefully and have consecrated it for the purpose of pure and simple meditation, contemplation, and prayer. Most of the music in this world has been poisoned by the energy of those who produced it. It has no place in your sacred spot, and God will not be with you if it is in competition with Him.

Your Mind Is The Altar of Your Body's Temple

Your body may be seated in your sacred spot, but your mind is where the sacrifice of silence and concentration is offered to God, possibly for the first time of your own conscious volition and pure motivation. The key to the true meaning of life lies in the awakening of the connection between your created spirit and the Creator Spirit, God.

Silence fosters prayer and meditation, and prayer and meditation form the channel through which you can center yourself and separate yourself from the material world so that you will be able to communicate directly with God, Who does not dwell in the material. There is a place inside everyone where the Spirit of God comes to visit in order to be in unity with the spirit of the human. Each person must rediscover that place and return to it.

Meditation and prayer is the vehicle that can transport a person's conscious awareness to that place of ultimate serenity and joy unlike anywhere on Earth. The process is simple and anyone can achieve success.

Meditation is widely practiced by people of all religions, and by those of no religion. It is the deliberate and intentional exercise of one's mind and spirit for the purpose of physical and mental relaxation and spiritual elevation. In our culture, it is often practiced and encouraged as a form of deep prayer for the purpose of communication and communion with God. Billy Graham has told his congregation that he meditates several hours each morning, and during his meditation time he communes deeply with God. St Teresa d'Avila meditated constantly. She called it her "prayer of quiet." Yogananda practiced and preached deep meditation all of his Earthly existence. Every great religious leader throughout history practiced meditation in one form or other during their lifetime.

In the New Testament, the Apostle Paul concludes his specific spiritual instructions to the disciple, Timothy, by telling him to *"Meditate upon these things; give thyself wholly to them."* (1 Timothy 4:15) He did not tell Timothy to sit in a lotus position, hold his fingers in the shape of a "mudra" and chant OM. He told him to meditate on what he had been taught by Paul—spiritual concepts of great importance.

In Genesis, Isaac, the son of Abraham, often *"went out to meditate in the field at eventide."* (Genesis 24:63) And he didn't do the chanting bit either. He was contemplating the teachings of his Faith, and he was talking to God. Meditation is not about you. Yes, it will help give you better health, but it is primarily about studying the teachings of God and talking to Him, so that you can invite His Presence into your entire life.

Meditation is encouraged throughout the Bible: Psalm 1:2, 19:14, 77:22, 107:43, 119:97; Proverbs 4:26; Joshua 1:8, for instance. When Jesus went into the wilderness for forty days, He went, in all probability, with the intention to spend those forty days in deep meditation with His Father in Heaven.

With the rise in interest in Eastern religions and New Age philosophies in the 1960s and 1970s, meditation came to be viewed by many as a foreign or heathen anti-Christian practice, self-centered in nature and having no value. More recently, however, attitudes have been shifting, bringing a better understanding of the practice of meditation, and of its role in a physically and spiritually healthy life. Many groups are forming within churches of all denominations for the purpose of meditative prayer, encouraged by the experience and insight of the church leaders. A Methodist pastor told me recently that meditation has completely changed how he prays to God; a Catholic church offers a meditation group that meets weekly in the fellowship hall to practice meditation on scripture verses and their central concepts; and a Baptist preacher confided that after years of narrow-mindedness, he now realizes that meditation is a way to pray deeply and sincerely. They are right; if done correctly and with proper intent, meditation will bring you closer to God than you ever thought possible.

How to Prepare for Meditation

There is no one, correct way to meditate, but there are a few things you can do in order to insure that your meditation session bears fruit. Following is a checklist of helpful tips you might wish to consider before beginning your own practice.

1. **Prepare your sacred spot for meditation**: As mentioned previously, it can be a closet, a screened-off corner of your bedroom, or the old trailer out back. This is essential. Keep the area clear of all material objects. Use it as a sanctuary and nothing else. Keep its energy centered on your spiritual practice alone. That energy will accumulate and remain in your spot as time goes by.

2. **Ensure quiet and solitude**: Put the dogs and cats outside and send the kids to the store (or anywhere) for the time you have allotted for your meditation or prayer. Unplug or turnoff all of the phones and put a "Do Not Disturb" sign on your door.

3. **Prepare your body:**
   - Wash your hands and face before you begin. Wear a set of clean, comfortable, loose-fitting clothes. Try to use the same clothes each time you meditate or pray, as simply the act of donning your "special clothes" will put your mind in the proper frame for meditation or prayer.
   - Before meditation, do 5-10 minutes of yoga asanas. I suggest Exalted Warrior, Cat-Cow, Triangle, Royal Pigeon, and Butterfly. These postures will limber you up and open your spine so that you will be more relaxed and receptive during your meditation time. These postures are described in detail in Chapter 7 as part of the complete sequence of Asanas.

- Do a Pranayama breathing exercise for about 5 minutes. Six complete **Spinal Breaths** as described at the end of this chapter is perfect. **The Circle of Joy** as described in Chapter 7 also works well for this purpose..
- Sit comfortably in a chair or cross-legged on the floor or on a cushion. It is not necessary to sit in a designated Yoga posture but do keep the body, head, and neck erect and straight, not slumped over or slouched. It is also important to remember that meditative consciousness rises upward along the path of the spine during its practice. A straight spine facilitates that flow, and by continuing the **spinal breathing** throughout the entirety of your session, your body will be reminded to maintain your erect posture.

4. **Prepare your mind:** Tell your mind to accept the fact that you are there for an important reason and for a specific duration of time. You have spent most of your day doing what the world wanted you to do, now you are going to spend just fifteen minutes (or whatever amount of time) doing what you and God want to do.

5. **Enter into your meditation:** Close your eyes and bring your attention to the space directly in front of your face. It isn't necessary to force your eyes to look upward, in fact, that practice can often defeat the purpose because it can be uncomfortable over an extended period of time. With your eyes closed, simply relax. Try to look deep into the darkness as if you were looking out into the deep night sky and just be silent. No mantras. No philosophical thoughts to ponder. No scripture verses to consider. Just *total silence*, and *listen* for God's Spirit communing with your own spirit. Meditation is about shutting out the world and listening to God. If you do this faithfully you will be surprised by what you will experience.

Try to meditate for 10 to 15 minutes a day at first, and work up gradually to a half hour or even an hour. Much of this will be dependent on your daily schedule, children, and other activities, of course. Meditation and prayer are sacred times for you to be in communication with God; what is more important than that? Most people spend far too much time doing worldly things and almost no time on being with God. No wonder the world is such a mess.

Meditation is much simpler than some would have you believe. Don't be too concerned if you experience difficulty in the initial stages. As you regularly sit in your Sacred Spot and give yourself over to the Spirit of God, you will find that it will become your favorite thing to do each day.

Meditation or prayer is not about personal enlightenment or "becoming holy." It is simply a time to bring quietness to your life so that you can talk to God. There are no strict, rigid rules to meditation. When you get right down to it, you don't even have to wear special clothes or have a special place as we talked about above. Those are suggestions for the beginner. God will listen to you anywhere if you are truly sincere about communicating with Him. The problem is that most people will not take the time to talk to God; everything else in their day is more important.

The only requirements for prayer and meditation are silence and you.

Spinal Breathing Exercise for Raising Awareness: a Form of Kriya Yoga

Close your eyes and inhale while you imagine warm energy rising from the bottom of your spine and traveling up the spine all the way to the top of your head. Keep your eyes closed and as you exhale, imagine the same warm energy traveling back down to the bottom of your spine. Do this very slowly 10 times in a row.

That is all there is to it! This is the spinal breathing technique used not just for a Kriya Yoga practice, but for every yoga session, meditation/prayer session, as well as any other activity having anything to do with spiritual development, religion, or health. It is also one of the most important things you will take away from this book. It may be *the* most important thing, as it is the secret solution to many problems facing mankind today.

You were probably taught to breathe (if you were taught at all) by visualizing the air traveling down into your lungs as you inhale by expanding your diaphragm, then traveling up and out of your lungs as you exhale. Stop doing that!

The key to proper, effective breathing is energy, not air. Imagine this instead: as you **inhale**, energy rises up your spine into the top of your head, and as you **exhale**, energy travels down your spine into your lower regions. Some like to visualize a little light (remember, light is energy) traveling upward with the inhalation and going back down with the exhalation.

As Carl Sagan so memorably told us, we are made of star-stuff. That means that every molecule of every cell in your body is directly connected to every star in all the created universes. By envisioning your breath this way, you will always be reminded of your eternal origins.

Truth is simple, all mankind needs to do is to learn how to breathe properly. After having read much this far, you will already be aware of just how important it is to breathe properly, just how much health it can bring to you, and just how much distress it can bring if you do not do it properly. Imagine an entire world of humans breathing with this meditative, healing form of stimulated, spinal rhythm. Think of the healing it would bring not only to the humans themselves, but also to the world of nature, a world that humans have been abusing for many centuries.

Use the spinal breathing technique for your meditation and prayer sessions, as well as your yoga asana sessions. At some point in the future you may even find that you use it every day as a matter of normal breathing. When you get to that point, you may also find many other wonderful, supernatural things happening within you.

7

The Asanas, or Postures

Probably the first thing that comes to mind with the mention of yoga is an image of a slim figure sitting, standing, reclining, or something in between with arms, legs, and torso bent, twisted, and intertwined in a stylistic pose. As you have discovered in the previous chapters, yoga is much more than just these postures. Practice of the asanas is, however, a central activity around which all other aspects of a yogic life can grow.

A quick search of the internet for "Yoga Asanas" brings up the Wikipedia page listing 256 separate postures of varying complexity and degrees of difficulty. Since this book is intended to be a basic handbook for living a yogic lifestyle, I am presenting a much shorter list of asanas of modest complexity and difficulty. Years of practice and teaching have proven this sequence of postures to be of maximum benefit to overall good health and well-being, and central to achieving and maintaining physical and spiritual vitality. Remember, true yoga is a formula dating back thousands of years. If practiced with unadorned simplicity the way the ancient yogins practiced it, the formula will work for you as well as it did for them. Altering the formula, or turning it into some form of Power Yoga, or Aerobics Yoga, or Hot Yoga, or whatever the current fad is, will not achieve the same results. H_2O without the O is not water; it's simply hydrogen gas. Add another oxygen, and H_2O becomes H_2O_2, hydrogen peroxide—definitely something you don't want to drink. The same is true for yoga; changing it in any way can make it ineffective or even harmful.

The following sequence of postures is all you need to begin and to maintain a yogic lifestyle. Each asana is named in Sanskrit and in English—including some alternate names you might find if you look them up—and is accompanied by step-by-step instructions with a photograph for visual reference. If you practice just these postures, you will have the complete formula; you will need nothing more.

Each posture provides a specific benefit for your body. By that I mean that every posture targets a specific part of the body. Each posture, especially when combined with proper breathing, exercises and cleanses the lungs and directs energy and nourishment to the associated life-support systems (circulatory, respiratory, muscular, nervous, endocrine, skeletal, digestive, etc.) A brief description of the particular benefits follows each asana.

You will find a list of a few common conditions and the asanas beneficial to each at the end of this chapter. If you have any of these problems, and you practice the corresponding asanas on a daily basis, you should experience noticeable relief within a few weeks, or even days.

> **DISCLAIMER**: *If you have or suspect that you have any chronic disease or health problem of any kind, ask your doctor before doing anything new to your body, including the following sequence of yoga postures. In addition, tell your yoga teacher of any physical problems you have before beginning a yoga class. Most instructors will work individually with their students in order to give them the most beneficial experience possible with their class.*

I am confident that your doctor will give you the okay on these postures, as they are easy to do and do not put strain on any part of your body. These are the same postures I have taught in my classes throughout my career, and I have never had any injuries in my classes. Not even one. On the contrary, I have had only positive reports of healings and even total cures of some maladies that have plagued my students throughout those years. In addition, my classes have been attended regularly by a number of local medical doctors, who also refer their patients to me for the therapeutic effects of consistent Yoga practice.

Yoga in general—and this sequence in particular—is a safe and enjoyable activity, but there are some things to keep in mind before you begin to ensure that your experience remains a good one.

First, keep your eyes open. Many of the asanas will challenge your sense of balance until you get used to them. You can avoid losing your balance by keeping your eyes open and softly focused on the middle distance. Don't be embarrassed to position yourself near a wall or piece of furniture that can be easily touched for added stability, if necessary.

If it hurts, don't do it. If you find that getting into the "ideal" position of an asana is painful, just relax, back off a bit, and readjust your position. Keep the image of the perfect pose in your mind as a guide, but listen to your body. If you are in a class, a good instructor will be sensitive to your requirements and will guide you gently into the best pose for you. Your instructor will also be able to advise you in the use of simple props such as a folded blanket, yoga blocks, or even a chair in order to gain maximum benefit without pain or injury. If you have an instructor who insists on forcing your body beyond its capacity, you need to leave the class and not go back. Yoga is not a competitive sport; it is a personal journey and a unique experience for each practitioner.

If you find the step-by-step instructions difficult to follow, refer to the illustrations for guidance. Remember, the picture is an ideal, *not an absolute*. Each body is unique in its needs and abilities, and your final form in each posture will reflect that. Every session will be rewarded with increased energy, well-being, and achievement.

Whether you are three years old or 103 years old, this gentle yoga sequence is within your abilities. The important thing is that you give it a try. If it helps you in body, mind or spirit, continue with it for a lifetime. It is my sincere hope that by following this yoga routine, you will experience the benefits that so many of my students already have.

Atma Jayam Yoga^{SM} Lifestyle Hatha Yoga Sequence

After you have made all your preparations—cleared a space, laid down your mat, changed into loose, comfortable clothing—take a few minutes to relax and let go of the day's tensions. Sit quietly in a cross-legged position on the floor. Take some deep, slow breaths as directed in the section on **spinal breathing** found at the end of **Chapter 6**. Begin the routine when your feel mind has calmed and your body has relaxed.

Stage One Warm-up

Circle of Joy
(3 repetitions)

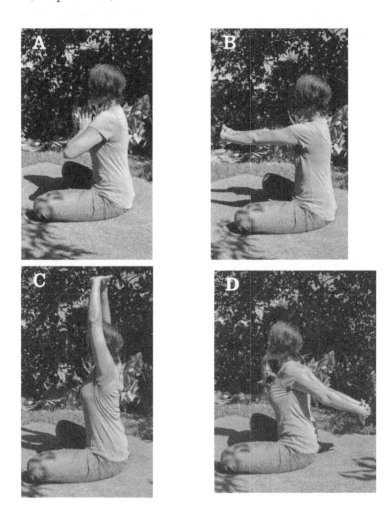

- Start in **Prayer Pose: Namaste (fig. A)**
  - Sit cross-legged on the floor.
  - Place the palms of your hands together in front of you, fingers together and pointed up (as if in prayer), elbows lifted to form a straight line from elbow through the wrists, to the other elbow.
- **Inhale** deeply and slowly while interlacing your fingers.
- **Exhale** slowly while pushing your hands out away from your chest, palms out, and fully extending your arms (**fig. B**).
- **Inhale** while raising your hands up in the air and over your head (**fig. C**).
- **Exhale** while unlacing your fingers. Bring your hands and arms down and behind you, level with the base of your spine. Interlace your fingers with your palms toward your body.
- **Inhale** as you extend your arms back behind you as far as you can that is comfortable (**fig. D**).
- **Exhale** as you unlace your fingers and bring your hands back around to the front of your body to the Namaste position.
- **Repeat** this sequence three times.

People who work in front of a computer all day need to take frequent breaks to rest the eyes and prevent the buildup of tension in muscles and joints. This sequence of stretching and deep breathing can be easily done while seated in a chair or while standing, and is great for relieving stress and tension throughout the workday.

Stage Two: The First Floor Sequence

Each of the following warm-up positions and Asanas should be held for thirty seconds to one minute after moving into the final position. You can gauge the time by counting your breath, with one inhale and one exhale counting as one breath. This practice is especially good for beginners, as they often concentrate on the form and movement and forget to breathe. Without the breath, yoga is just a pose. Your mind makes a stronger connection with your body when you focus your attention by counting your breaths, enhancing the benefits of the particular posture.

You can hold any of these postures for as long as you like, but for maximum effect, that should be at least thirty seconds. Conversely, while it will do no harm to go longer than one minute, there is nothing to be gained from the asanas in this sequence by remaining in position longer. The exceptions to this advice are any inversion postures, or those that place the level of the head below that of the heart; these should be held for thirty seconds or less, depending on the extremity of the inversion.

Be sure to rest between each posture for 10–5 seconds—two or three deep breaths—before starting the next one.

2.1 Corpse or Relaxation: Savasana

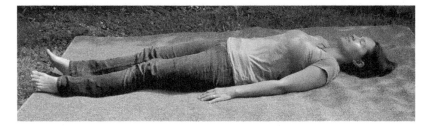

Yes, this really is a yoga asana.

- Lie flat on your back with your arms to your side, with your eyes open or closed, and relax.

2.2 Hip Openers (2 repetitions)

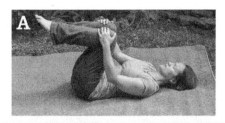

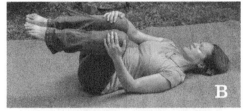

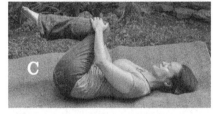

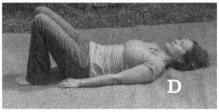

- Lift your feet off the floor and bring your knees toward your chest (**12:00; fig. A**). Do not pull your knees toward you; let their own weight do the work.
- Rock to the left just a couple of inches (knees at 10:00; fig. B) and relax the right hip for about 30 seconds.
- Rock to the right until your knees are at 2:00 (**fig. C**), and relax the left hip for 30 seconds.
- Repeat the last two movements.
- Return knees to the 12:00 position and place your feet flat on the floor with your heels close to your buttocks (**fig. D**).

2.3 Knee Drops

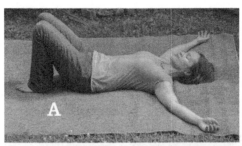

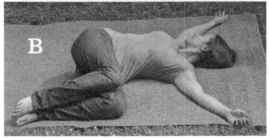

- Extend your arms straight out from your shoulders, palms facing up (**fig. A**).
- Allow your knees to drop to your left toward the floor as far as is comfortable (**fig. B**).
  - Your feet will not be flat on the floor, but both should be in contact with it.
- Relax in this position for about one minute. Return to the starting position.
- Repeat the movement to the right. Relax for one minute, and then return to the starting position (**Hip Openers, fig. D**).
- Take a deep breath in and out.

Note: If you suffer from stiffness and/or pain in your back and hips, try doing the hip opener and knee drops first thing in the morning. Just throw your covers back and do them on the bed before getting up.

2.4 Bridge: Setsu Bandhasana

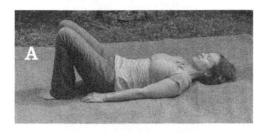

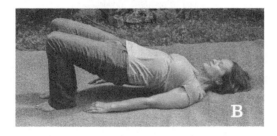

- Position your arms parallel to your body with the palms facing down. Make sure that your feet are flat on the floor, and your knees are up and your legs are parallel to each other from your ankles to your knees (**fig. A**).
- Using your shoulders, arms and hands, and feet as anchors, raise your buttocks off the floor as high as is comfortable (**fig. B**).
- Hold the raised position for thirty seconds to one minute, breathing slowly and deeply.
- Return to the start position.
- Rise into a cross-legged sitting position (carefully to avoid dizziness) with your hands resting palm up on your knees in preparation for the next pose.

Note: The Bridge Pose relieves stress in the muscles of the back, and stretches and tones the muscles of the neck, chest and spine.

2.5 Seated Heron (or Swan)

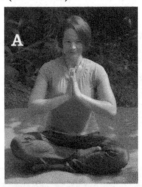

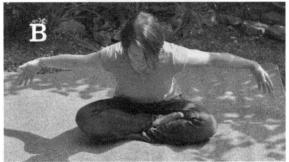

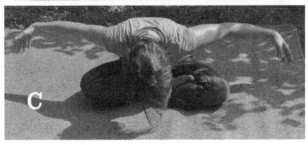

- Bring hands and arms to the **Prayer** or **Namaste** position (**fig. A**).
- **Inhale** deeply.
- **Exhale** slowly while opening your arms wide, dropping them slightly while relaxing your wrists and hands (**fig. B**).
  - Each of your arms should form a gentle arc from shoulder to fingertip; elbows below and a little behind the shoulders, hands forward and below elbows, wrists limp so that your hands dangle loosely with your fingertips between waist level and the floor.

- Lean forward. Keep your back straight and allow your head to fall toward your chest—just relax and let gravity do the work for thirty seconds to a minute (**fig. C**).
- Return to **Namaste** position and pause before continuing.

Note: The key to this pose is to imagine that your body is a limp form draped on a ridged frame—like a scarecrow hanging on a pole. This is a very relaxing posture, and is excellent for relieving tension in the neck and for lengthening the spine.

Stage Three: The Standing Sequence

General Instructions

Standing Mountain: Tadasana

This is the "home" position for the standing sequences.

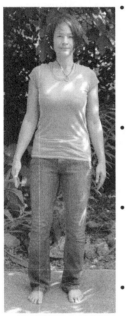

- Stand with your feet as close together as possible while maintaining your balance. Keep your feet parallel by making sure that the second and middle toes of each foot are pointing straight ahead. Feel your body make solid contact with the floor evenly through the soles of your feet.
- Keep your knees slightly bent or straight, but *not* locked. Be aware of the muscles in your calves and thighs as they actively engage in keeping your balance.
- Feel a line of energy running up from the base of your spine to the top of your head, straightening your spine and aligning your neck so that your chin is parallel to the floor.
- Shoulders are level and straight, with your arms hanging relaxed at your sides.

The first posture, **Moon Pose**, is center oriented and done once in this sequence.

The next three standing postures are done as a single fluid motion focusing first on the left side of the body. After returning to the center, **Standing Mountain (Tadasana)**, for a brief pause, the postures will be repeated, focusing on the right side of the body, and returning to **Tadasana**.

3.1 Moon Pose: Chandrasana

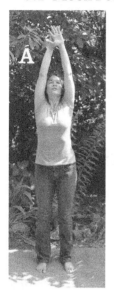 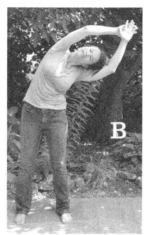 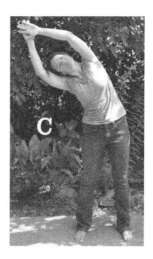

- Begin in **Standing Mountain.**
- While **inhaling** slowly
  - Raise your arms straight from each side until they extend straight up from each shoulder (**fig. A**).
  - With palms facing forward, bring your hands together over your head, placing the back of one hand in the palm of the other.
- While **exhaling** slowly
  - Stretch the right side of your body so that your body curves to the left (**fig. B**).
  - Your raised hands will move from 12 o'clock to 11 or 10 o'clock.
  - Keep your weight even on both feet, shifting your hips and pelvis as little as possible.
  - Your body will resemble a crescent moon.
  - Hold the position for up to a minute.
- **Inhale** while returning to 12 o'clock, then, without pausing
- **Exhale** while stretching the left side of your body so that your body curves to the right (**fig. C**).

3.1 Moon Pose, continued
  - Your raised hands will move from 12 o'clock to 1 or 2 o'clock.
  - Keep your weight even on both feet, shifting your hips and pelvis as little as possible.
  - Your body will resemble a crescent moon.
  - Hold the position for up to a minute.
- **Inhale** while returning to 12 o'clock.
- **Exhale** while returning to **Standing Mountain**.

Note: The overhead stretch opens up the chest and draws breath into areas of the lungs normally not fully engaged in breathing. This posture also stretches the spine, opening up space between the vertebrae. The Moon Pose is an ideal exercise to do during a short work break. The full-body stretch and enhanced breathing is energizing, and requires very little space; it can even be done while seated.

3.2 Warrior 2: Virabhadrasana 2

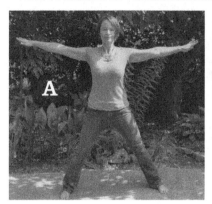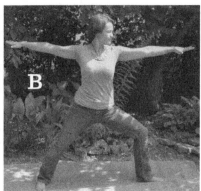

- From **Standing Mountain,** increase the distance between your feet so that your legs form a triangle with the floor; a distance about equal to the length of your leg.
- Raise your arms straight up from each side to shoulder height (**fig. A**).
- Keeping your right leg and foot stationary, rotate your left leg so that the foot is turned 90° left.
- Bend your left knee while keeping your right leg straight.
  - Keep your knee centered over your heel and your shin perpendicular to the floor.
  - You can adjust the amount of stretch you feel in your groin by moving your right foot closer to or further from your left foot.
  - **CAUTION:** Do not allow your knee to move forward of your heel, as this can cause stress or injury.
- Turn your head to look out over the fingers of your left hand.
  - Arms and shoulders are straight across from fingertip to fingertip.
  - Chest, hips, and right leg and foot all face forward.
  - Left foot, knee, and leg align with the left arm and head. (**fig. B**).
- Hold for 30 seconds, and then continue to **Warrior 1.**

Note: The Warrior 2 posture and the Warrior 1 posture that follows work to strengthen your quadriceps (the front of your thigh.) They are also what are termed "empowering" postures. As you place yourself into either of the postures, imagine that you are a mighty warrior. These are great to do when you are at work just after the boss chews you out—or when you are at home and the kids say, "Vegeburgers again!"

3.3 Warrior 1: Vibrahadrasana 1

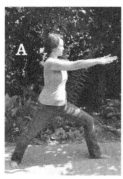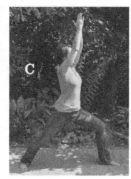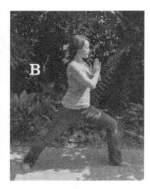

- Starting from the final position of **Warrior 2**, bring your right hand around to meet your left, palms together. **(fig. A)**
  - Your hips and shoulders will reorient to the same direction as your left foot, leaving your right leg extended behind you, with the right foot pointed 90° right.
  - Your left knee will still be bent.
  - DO NOT allow your knee to extend beyond your ankle!
- Draw your hands to your chest into the prayer position **(fig. B)**.
- Keep your palms together and continue the movement by extending your arms above your head (**fig. C**).
  - If your neck muscles are strong, tip your head back and follow the motion of your arms with your eyes. If you have any problems with this head position—weakness, pain, dizziness, etc.—just keep your head level and look straight ahead.
- Hold for 30 seconds.
- Return to **position B**, inhaling deeply before continuing to Standing Swan.

3.4 Standing Heron (or Swan)

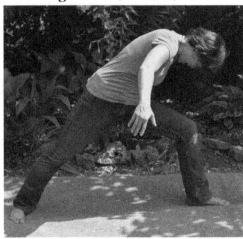
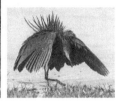

- From the final position of **Warrior 1**, exhale slowly as you lower your hands to the prayer position.
- Continue the motion as you did in **Seated Heron**.
    - Open your arms wide to resemble spread wings, extending them back a bit and letting them drop while relaxing your wrists and hands, forming a gentle arc from one fingertip, through the shoulders, to the other fingertip.
    - Let your hands hang loosely from your wrists at about the level of your hips and a little behind them.
- Lean forward over your extended leg. Keep your back straight but relax your neck so that your chin drops toward your chest. (**see figure above**)
    - **Pay attention to the position of your knee and ankle!**
- Hold the position for 30 seconds.
- Return to **Standing Mountain**.
    - Raise your head and torso, and lower your arms.
    - Straighten your left leg, rotating it and your hips and shoulders to face forward.
- Bring your feet together to finish in **Standing Mountain**. Rest in this position for 10 to 15 seconds (two or three deep breaths).

Repeat Warrior 2, Warrior 1, and Standing Heron.

- In **Warrior 2** instructions, substitute RIGHT for LEFT.
- Movements in **Warrior 1** and **Standing Heron** will follow in this direction.
- Finish in **Standing Mountain,** and rest for 10 to 15 seconds before proceeding

3.5 Triangle Pose (Trikonasana) with an Extra Side Stretch.

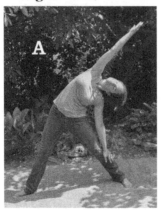 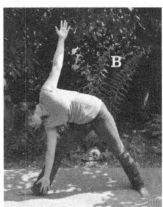

- Raise your arms to each side to shoulder height, parallel to the floor, palms facing downward.
- Move your feet wide apart—the distance about equal to the length of your leg.
- If you have trouble keeping your balance, move your feet together until you are more stable.
- Turn your right foot out so that your toes point in the same direction as the fingers of your right hand.
- Turn your head so that you are looking out over your right hand.
- Keeping your arms straight across the shoulders, tip your torso to the left as far as possible, bending sideways rather than forward or back.
  - Your right arm will rise toward the ceiling, as your left arm drops toward the floor (**fig. A**).
  - Imagine that your body is a bow with the string fastened to the top of your head and your left foot. The bow (your body) is gathering energy as the string is being pulled to launch the arrow.
  - Make your right side as long as possible by stretching your body straight from your fingertips, expanding your ribs, and lifting them up and away from your pelvis.
  - This stretch will be similar to the stretch you did in the **Moon** pose.

- Release the arrow. Flex back to the right, through the center, and continue as far as is comfortable (**fig. B**).
  - **Arm position**
    - ○ Your right arm is down, and your left arm is up. Keep a straight line across your fingertips, arms and shoulders.
  - The arm positions may be modified as follows for comfort.
    - ○ Hold your left arm out straight from your shoulder, or bend your elbow, placing your hand on your left hip.
    - ○ Rest your right hand on your left leg at a point that is comfortable, above or below, but not on your knee.
  - **Head position**
    - ○ The "perfect" position is to turn your head to look up at your left hand. This position is also awkward and potentially dangerous.
    - ○ The SAFE position is to look straight ahead or down at the floor.
- Remember to breathe while you hold the position for 30 seconds to one minute.
- Slowly straighten your torso and lower your arms.
- Reverse the position of your feet, and repeat the movements in the opposite direction.
- Finish in **Standing Mountain,** and rest for 10 to 15 seconds

Note: This posture, as well as **Warrior 1 and Warrior 2,** opens up and strengthen the spine and lower back. The **Triangle** also strengthens virtually all of the muscles of your torso, refining your waist, abdomen, back and chest. In addition, it stretches your hamstrings, opens up the lungs, strengthens and stimulates the kidneys, and stimulates and heals the male prostate gland. Maintaining the position of the arms and shoulders throughout this asana aids in relieving carpal tunnel syndrome. Regular practice of this posture also strengthens the muscles and support structure of the hips, reducing the risk of fracture with aging.

3.6 Flute Player Pose: a variation of the Tree Pose (Vrksasana)

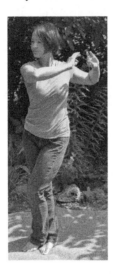 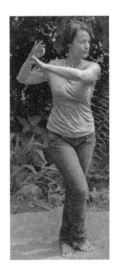

- **Inhale** deeply, and **exhale** slowly.
- Arm position
  - Imagine yourself playing the flute
  - Lift both elbows away from your body so the your upper arm extends at a 45° angle from your shoulder.
  - Raise both hands straight up from your elbows, palms facing forward, fingers relaxed and slightly curled.
  - Swing your right arm from the shoulder across your chest, raising your elbow somewhat, so that your right hand is between your left hand and your head. Your right palm will now face back while your left remains facing forward.
- Feet and legs:
  - Cross your left in front of your right.
  - Place your left foot next to your right, little toe to little toe, leaving the left heel elevated.
  - Feel your weight evenly through your entire right foot and the ball and toes of your left.
- Head:
  - Turn your head to the right and down a little. You will be looking at the floor about six feet beyond and slightly to the right of your right elbow.

- Keep your eyes open.
- Hold for 30 seconds to one minute before returning to center Standing Mountain.
- Repeat the posture to the right.

Note: This is a balance posture so leave your eyes open as you do this. If you have serious balance issues do not cross one leg in front of the other, but remain standing with your legs straight and parallel. You will still get the same benefits from the pose without the more difficult balance. Your stability in this pose will improve with practice. As it does, you can begin to move your feet and legs into the more challenging position.

The benefits of the **Flute Player** include improved balance and strengthening of the lower back, upper spine, and neck.

This posture seems complicated, but with practice you will be able to perform it as one smooth movement. As with all of the asanas, refer to the illustrations for clarification.

3.7 Lightning Bolt Pose: Utkatasana, also known as "Chair" or "Thunderbolt"

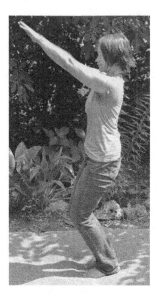

- Begin in **Standing Mountain Pose** either with feet together, or for better balance, feet separated up to hip-distance.
- **Inhale** and raise your arms in front of you, any where from shoulder height to just forward of your ears, depending on your strength.
- **Exhale** as you bend your knees as if you are going to sit on a chair.
  - Keep your back straight as your hips move back to "find the chair."
  - Keep your feet flat.
  - Keep your weight over your heels as much as possible.
  - Don't let your knees go forward beyond your toes. Check by looking down in front of your knees. If you can't see your toes, adjust the angle of you hips and pelvis until you can.
- Keeping your head level, direct your gaze upward.
  - Breath normally while holding this position for up to one minute.

- **Inhale** as you stand up straight.
- **Exhale** as you lower your arms and return to **Standing Mountain**

Note: This pose builds strength and stability in the feet, ankles, and legs. It also strengthens the lower back and abdomen.

3.8 Jackknife Diver Pose: a variation of Padahastasana, also known as "Standing Forward Fold"

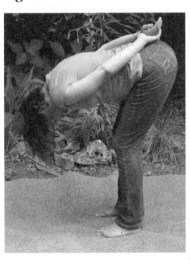

- Begin in **Standing Mountain,** with your feet positioned for maximum balance.
- Bring your hands behind you and place them palms up, one on top of the other, over your sacrum at the base of your spine.
  - This placement will remind you to keep your spine straight rather than curved, and your shoulders back instead of rounded as you fold forward, thus protecting the muscles of your lower back from strain.
- **Inhale** deeply.
- **Exhale** as you bend forward from your hips.
  - Bend only as far as you can without forcing yourself.
  - Keep your knees straight but not locked.
  - Relax your neck and allow your head to drop forward. You are not striving to reach the floor, but gently folding your chest and belly toward your thighs.
  - If you have high blood pressure, keep your head above the level of your hips.

- Hold the position for up to a minute.
  - Breath normally.
  - Use each inhalation to lift and lengthen your torso, and each exhalation to relax deeper into the pose while keeping your spine straight.
- Bring your hands forward and use them to help position yourself on your hands and knees for the **Table Pose.**
  - If you choose to stand up straight rather than continue to the **Table Pose,** do so carefully to avoid dizziness.

Note: If you have a heart condition or high blood pressure, keep your head at or above the level of your hips. A similar stretch for the neck, back and legs can be attained by doing this posture as a seated forward fold without the risk of it becoming an inverted posture.

People with lower back pain or spinal problems should also avoid the **Jackknife Diver.** Consult your doctor to help determine the limits of your abilities and the weakness you need to be aware of. Your instructor can then help you with variations of this (or any other) pose that will address your unique issues.

Four: Second Floor Routine

4.1 Table Pose

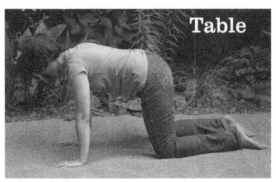

- Place your hands on the floor squarely below your shoulders with your fingers facing forward.
  - A folded towel may be used to relieve pressure on sensitive knees.
  - If you need to relieve the pressure on your wrists, make fists with your hands and rest your weight on your knuckles, keeping your wrists straight. You may need to play around a bit to get the right position for your comfort.
- Position your knees directly under your hips so that your thighs are perpendicular to the floor.
  - Your lower legs will extend straight back from your knees, and the tops of your feet will be against the floor, causing your toes to point.
  - Your back is flat, your neck is straight, and you are looking at the floor between your hands.
  - Do not let your belly drop.

Note: This simple and relaxing posture strengthens the wrists, arms, and shoulders. It also tones the muscles of the back and abdomen, while expanding the chest and improving lung capacity.

4.2 Cat-Cow

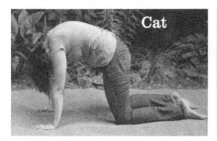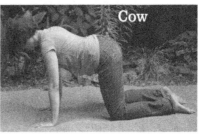

- While in **Table Pose, inhale** deeply.
- **Cat**
  - While **exhaling** as much air as possible, arch your back upwards, pulling your belly button up toward your spine.
  - Relax your neck and allow your chin to tuck in toward your chest.
- **Cow**
- While **inhaling**, drop your belly toward the floor.
  - Lift your head, chin, and chest, letting your back to curve downward.
  - Start the movement at the base of the spine and let it roll up your back to your neck and head.
- Repeat the sequence as many times as you like.
  - Move slowly and purposefully, exhaling into the arched-back Cat and inhaling into the sway-backed Cow.
- Come to rest in **Table Pose**

Note: The simple combination of postures and breathing that comprise **Cat-Cow** is one of the best in yoga. The gentle flexion and extension of the spine keep it supple and relaxed through the day, reducing the occurrence of spinal problems. The deep breathing is invigorating and brings healing and refreshment to the entire body. The **Cat-Cow** can also be done at work while seated at your desk.

- Sit up straight on the front edge of the seat of your chair.
- Position your chair so that your arms are straight when you place them on your desk.
- Place your feet flat on the floor.
- Proceed with the movements and breathing of **Cat-Cow**, doing as many repetitions as you like.

Now, don't you feel better?

If you were to choose only two yoga postures to do faithfully every day, this would be one of them. The other would be the **Circle of Joy** described at the beginning of the sequence. There is incredible healing and vitality in just those two postures. Remember, when you approach yoga as if you are "eating" nutrition and health, it can become a Fountain of Youth for you.

4.3 Balancing Table

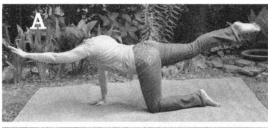

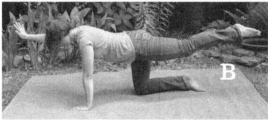

- Start in **Table Pose** with your back flat, belly tight, hands directly under your shoulders, knees directly under your hips, your head level, and your gaze directed to a point between your hands (this will help keep you stable).
- **Inhale** and raise your RIGHT knee, bringing it forward slightly, then extending your leg straight out behind you parallel to the floor, if you can, but not higher than your shoulders.
- **Exhale** as you stabilize yourself in this position.
- Keeping your right leg extended, **inhale** as you lift your LEFT arm straight forward at shoulder height. Extend your body from right fingertips to left toes (**fig. A**).
- Hold the position for five or six deep breaths.
- **Exhale** as you lower your leg and arm and return to **Table Pose**.
- Rest for two or three breaths, then repeat the posture with the opposite leg and arm (**fig. B**).

Note: This asana builds core strength and improves balance. While it appears to be quite simple, it requires focus and concentration to master this pose. You may want to work up to it by raising one arm or leg at a time. Another beginner trick is to extend the leg but keep the toes of that foot in contact with the floor. With practice you will soon develop the strength and balance to elevate your leg while extending the opposing arm.

4.4 Royal Pigeon: Rajakapotasana, Sleeping Pigeon variation

Practice this asana carefully, one step at a time.

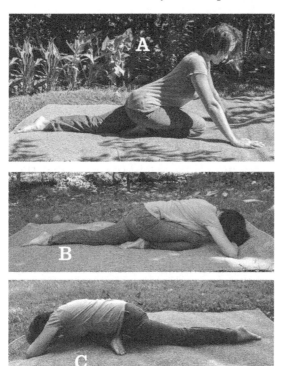

- Start in **Table Pose**
- Bring your right knee forward and place it on the mat in line with your right hip while keeping your left leg straight behind you.
    - Keep your hips level and squared as this movement lowers your body.
    - If there is tightness in the hip of your forward leg, keep your foot positioned directly under that thigh, as can be seen in **figure A**.
    - If you are more flexible, then flex your foot and CARE-FULLY move it forward, away from your body while keeping your knee pointing straight ahead (as can be seen in **figure C**).

4.4 Pigeon, continued

CAUTION: *If you feel any pain or pressure in your knee, stop and return to the original position.*

- Bend forward from your hips, extending your upper body over your right leg.
    - Use your hands to carry your weight as you "walk" them forward.
- Position your torso in the position you find most comfortable, using your hands or forearms as props (**fig. A**).
    - You can continue to lower your upper body so that you are resting folded over your extended right thigh (**fig. B and C**).
- Keep your weight balanced between both hips.
- Hold the position for up to a minute, breathing deeply.
- Carefully return to **Table Pose**.
    - Use your hands to "walk" your body back into position.
    - Move with care to avoid torsion and strain on knees and hips.
- Repeat steps 1–6, bringing the left knee forward and extending the right leg back.

Note: The benefits of this asana are almost infinite. Everything including hips, groin, hamstrings, quadriceps, chest, shoulders, lungs, and lower back, is stretched, stimulated and strengthened by it. It is particularly helpful for relief from sciatic pain; a number of my students over the years have been able to eliminate it entirely with daily practice of this posture.

4.5 Butterfly: Baddha Konasana, also known as "Cobbler Pose"

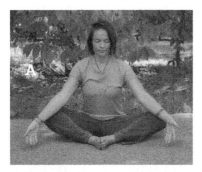
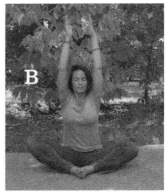
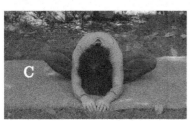

- Assume a seated position with your spine straight, your legs outstretched, and your hands at your side on the mat.
- Bend your knees and draw your feet toward your body.
- Press the soles of your feet together and allow your knees to drop open naturally. DO NOT press on your knees to open them further, as this could cause injury.
- Rest your hands lightly in a comfortable spot on your feet or legs, keeping your spine straight and your weight balanced (**fig. A**).
- **Inhale** while raising your arms out to each side, then straight up from the shoulders (**fig. B**).
- **Exhale** as you fold forward from the hips, keeping your arms extended and your back straight.
- When you have folded as far as you can without forcing yourself, let your arms relax and drape in front of you (**fig. C**).
- Tuck in your chin and relax your neck.
- Hold the posture for at least a minute, breathing deeply and relaxing further with each exhalation.

4.5 Butterfly, Continued

- Slowly return to the upright position, bringing your hands together as in **Namaste**.
- Pause for 30 to 60 seconds, then continue to **Savasana with Elevated Knees**

Note: Very few people can fold completely so that their chest is lying on their thighs. Don't worry about it; go as far as you can and let gravity do its work. The important thing to remember is that you are folding forward from your hips, not rolling up from your shoulders. Let your arms, neck, and hips relax while you keep your spine straight and your shoulders back.

4.6 Savasana with Elevated Knees

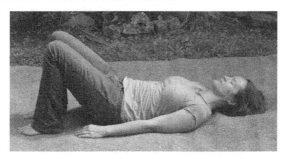

- Lie on your back with your arms at your sides, parallel to your body.
- **Inhale**, then **exhale** deeply.
- Keeping your feet together, place them flat on the floor, and draw them toward your body to comfortably elevate your knees.
- Hold this posture for a minute or so, breathing normally.

Note: This simple inversion posture is good for relaxing blood flow and lowering blood pressure

4.7 Dying Bug

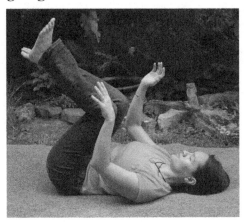

- Begin in **Savasana with elevated knees.**
- Keeping your knees bent, lift your feet from the floor. Let gravity do the work of separating your knees and pulling them toward your chest.
- Keeping your wrists and elbows somewhat loose, bring your arms up over your torso.
- Wiggle your body while waving your arms and legs above you, like a bug on it's back, or a dog scratching it's back on a carpet.
- Return your feet to the floor, extend your legs, and position your arms in **Savasana.**

4.8 Savasana with Progressive relaxation

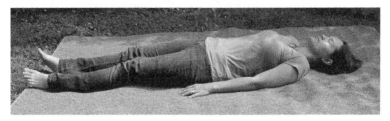

- Lie quietly in **Savasana** for up to a minute.
- Tense and relax the muscles in each part of your body in turn, starting with your feet and working up:
  - feet
  - calves
  - thighs
  - buttocks
  - stomach
  - hands and forearms
  - upper arms and biceps
  - chest
  - neck
  - face
- **Inhale** as you tense, and **exhale** as you relax each muscle group.
- Close your eyes and lie in **Savasana** for 2 to 5 minutes of total relaxation.
- Return to the moment
- Take a deep breath in and out.
- Wiggle your toes and fingers for a few seconds.
- Turn your head from side to side slowly 2 or 3 times.
- Stretch out your arms and legs.
- Take a deep breath, yawning if you need to.
- Open your eyes and sit up slowly.
  - Most people acknowledge the end of the session with a quiet "Namaste," or "Praise God."

And that is the end of the entire routine.

Daily practice of this yoga sequence will result in improved physical, mental, and spiritual health for a lifetime.

A reminder of the cautions from the beginning of the routine:

1. **If you find the step-by-step instructions difficult to follow, refer to the illustrations for guidance.**
   - Every body is different. If you *imagine* yourself taking the pose in the picture, your body will do its best to follow. The results will be close enough.
2. **If it hurts, DON'T DO IT.**
   - See explanation of point one above.
3. **Keep your eyes open.**

There are many other yoga asanas you can learn to add to or vary this routine, but that's not really necessary. I created this simple routine many years ago specifically for the purpose of enhancing health and well-being, not for exercise, aerobics, or sport—as many of today's yoga classes seem to be—and it WORKS.

In my many years of practicing and teaching yoga I have had numerous doctors and healthcare practitioners take my classes, verifying that practice of this routine is beneficial, and if done with care and as directed, will do no harm. Not only do doctors attend my classes, but they send their patients as well.

A Short List of Disorders and Recommended Asanas

- **Arthritis**:
  - All of the postures in the sequence are good for nearly all forms of arthritis. Don't worry about perfection; hold the image of the posture in your mind and let your body do as well as it can. A good instructor can assist you with adaptations and the use of props to make the most of your practice.
- **Asthma**:
  - Jackknife Diver, Bridge
- **Brain and Memory**:
  - Cat-Cow, Jackknife Diver, and most of the other postures. Most forms of dementia can be traced to either circulatory issues, or blocked systems in the body (especially the spine.) The entire Yoga sequence and these postures especially address these issues.
- **Blood Circulation and General Health**:
  - The entire routine
- **Common Cold**:
  - The entire routine
- **Chronic Fatigue**:
  - The entire routine
- **Diabetes**:
  - Triangle, Cat-Cow, Circle of Joy
- **Digestion**:
  - Moon, Triangle
- **Spine and Discs**:
  - Triangle, Cat-Cow, and all other postures
- **Eyes**:
  - Lightning Bolt, Cat-Cow, Circle of Joy
- **Fibromyalgia**:
  - The entire routine
- **Headaches, including Migraines**:
  - The entire routine, but especially the Cat-Cow.

- **Knees**:
  - Moon, Lightning Bolt
- **Lower Back**:
  - Triangle, Jackknife Diver, Cat-Cow
- **Lungs**: (See also asthma)
  - The entire routine
- **Multiple Sclerosis**:
  - The entire routine
- **Mammary Glands**:
  - Cat-Cow, Circle of Joy
- **Neck**:
  - The entire routine
- **Nervous System, Depression**:
  - The entire routine, but especially the Triangle
- **Prostate**
  - Triangle
- **Sciatic Nerve Problems**:
  - Royal Pigeon, Jackknife Diver, Cat-Cow
- **Sexual Problems**:
  - The entire routine
- **Shoulders**:
  - Triangle, Moon
- **Spine**:
  - The entire routine
- **Thyroid**:
  - The entire routine

8

A Summary of the Yogic Lifestyle

This chapter is a summary of the practices and principles that
are a part of every yogi's life, from the raw beginner to the seasoned
and venerable Yogiraj, or Master of Yoga. Use it as a quick reference
to remind yourself of the physical, mental and spiritual practices
that form the core of the Yogic lifestyle leading to physical health
and mental and spiritual well-being.

Moderation in All Things

Moderation is a word that has appeared many times throughout this book, and for good reason. While most people these days
realize that the practice of yoga does not require one to sleep naked
on a bed of nails, to never cut their hair or fingernails, or to meditate
twenty-three hours a day, there is still the idea that yoga is an austere
lifestyle of rigorous physical exercise, strict dietary constraints, and
demanding mental and spiritual discipline. Nothing could be further
from the truth. Yoga is the science of moderation and balance in
life, for the purpose of reaching regular communion with God.

The principle of ahimsa (do no harm) might lead you to consider being a vegetarian, but that is not required. What is necessary is
that your consumption of *everything* you eat is subject to self-control
(tapas), and that you acknowledge and respect the source.

While there are scientific studies suggesting that consuming
small amounts of alcohol on a regular basis — one or two per day,
three or four times per week, depending on your size, sex, age, and
general health — contributes to good health, there is a fine distinction between enough and too much, with the consequences of too
much being far worse than those of none or not enough. Of greater
concern than the physical effects of alcohol are its effects on the
mind and spirit. Alcohol numbs and confuses the mind, causing one
to lose self-control, and the after effects of over consumption result
in the depression of the spirit. If you choose to consume alcoholic

beverages once in a while, do so carefully and conscientiously.

We live in a finite physical world while striving to establish and maintain a connection with the infinite spiritual world, which means that the yamas of aparigraha (don't be greedy) and the niyama of santosha (practice contentment) are constantly being challenged. You do need a roof over your head and clothes to wear, but use moderation when making your choices—a simple house; adequate clothing. Find the balance between your wants (greed) and your needs (contentment).

Life is a dynamic process. All aspects of life—physiological functions, achieving and maintaining physical strength and stability, emotions, establishment of proper relationships with other people, functioning in a material world while maintaining an awareness of and a presence in the Spiritual world—are subjected to constantly shifting opposing forces that must be kept in balance. Moderation in all things—a primary key to a yogic lifestyle—will allow you to do just that.

Asanas

Spend time each day doing yoga postures. Many of you have jobs that generate mental and physical tensions that need to be released throughout the day. A five-minute break each hour will alleviate the stress and avoid much of the pain, injury, and illness that it can cause. Many of the asanas can be modified to fit the confines of a small office or cubicle, and are particularly suited to relieve the tension that builds up in the neck, back, shoulders, and arms. Alternate these mini-yoga sessions with a walk down the hall and back every hour or so, and add in some deep breathing during the day; you will find that you will have accomplished more work and that you are more alert at the end of the day than ever before.

Devote thirty minutes to an hour once or twice a week or more to focus on the complete series of yoga postures. It is advantageous if at least one of those sessions is with an instructor in a class. A trained and certified yoga teacher can guide your form and movement so that you will experience the maximum benefit and avoid potential injury. The formal setting of a class and the commitment to attend will give you added incentive to continue on your chosen path, even if your resolve begins to weaken when you are on your own. The class also becomes a community of like-minded individuals with whom you can share experiences and insights.

Pranayama

Yogic breathing is the catalyst that activates the combined elements of yoga. This conscientious and energizing inhalation and exhalation of breath can be your Fountain of Youth.

Pay close attention to the breathing exercises performed during yoga asana sessions, as proper breathing enhances the benefits of the postures. Ask your teacher to instruct you in some of the variations of pranayama not covered in this book, such as Sudarsan Kriya, Nadi Shodhanam, Bhastrika Pranayama, among others. Our friend, The Internet, can fill you in on their details, purpose, and application. For your everyday practice however, simple **spinal breathing** as described in Chapter 6 is all you need.

Meditation and Prayer

A true yogin meditates and/or prays at least twice a day. The best times for meditation are early in the morning and in the evening before you go to bed.

Spend at least fifteen minutes once or twice each day in order to realize improvements in health such as stress relief, lowering of blood pressure, relief of arthritic back and joint pain, etc. By extending at least one of the daily sessions to an hour or more, you will be rewarded with increased personal and spiritual insight, especially if it follows a series of asanas and pranayama.

Meditation is like running a marathon; you don't get up one day and run twenty-six miles, you work up to it. When you first begin to practice meditation, don't expect to last more than fifteen minutes before you start to fidget and the outside world invades your tranquility. Don't be discouraged. Each time you meditate you will find more mental and spiritual avenues to explore and more ways to block out the worldly distractions, gradually extending the time you spend in meaningful contemplation. After a while — maybe three months to a year—the fifteen minutes that seemed like an eternity will become an hour that seems like no time at all.

Diet

Here, too, let moderation be your guide to achieving the balance between your wants and your needs. Find contentment by eating slowly and savoring every bite; don't give in to greed by rapidly consuming everything in sight.

So if moderation is the ideal, how does fasting fit in? Fasting is a regular part of the yogic path, conferring both physical and spiritual rewards.

It doesn't take much; just twenty-four hours ingesting nothing but water once a week, or once or twice a month. If that seems daunting, start out by just skipping a meal. When mealtime rolls around again, have a glass of water—I find that room temperature or warm (not hot) filtered or spring water tends to be the most satisfying—and see if you can make it to the next mealtime. Keep yourself occupied with light physical activities such as yoga asanas, meditation or prayer, reading, or anything as long as it is not too strenuous. The time will pass quickly, and you will have successfully completed your first fast.

The physiological benefits of regular fasting are well documented and can be summarized broadly as giving your body a chance to cleanse itself of toxins and reset its metabolism. Of equal or even greater significance are the mental and spiritual benefits to be gained. Even a limited fast; that is, consuming limited quantities of whole fruits or fruit juices, whole vegetables or vegetable juices, or broth, provides a cleansing pause in your daily routine during which the concern of want versus need can be objectively considered. When you return to your normal diet, it will be with new insight and sense of balance where food is concerned.

Karma Yoga

Karma can be thought of most simply as the spiritual law of cause and effect. The concept has been around almost since the beginning of time, and is expressed in the Bible by these verses:

> *7 Do not be deceived: God cannot be mocked. A man reaps what he sows. 8 Whoever sows to please their flesh, from flesh will reap destruction; whoever sows to please the Spirit, from the Spirit will reap eternal life. 9 let us not become weary in doing good, for at the proper time we will reap a harvest if we do not give up.*
> Galatians 6:7-9 (NIV)

Modern thought has reduced the concept of karma to the phrase, "What goes around, comes around."

Nearly all spiritual traditions use the promise of punishment or reward in some future life as inducement for doing good in this one. Even for those who are not particularly spiritually minded, there is a strong sense that the good or bad that is done in the present will have some effect on one's future fortunes.

The promise of reward or punishment is a strong motivator while establishing the pattern for a life of good works, but karma yoga elevates that chosen life to an even higher plane. A yogin practicing karma yoga seeks to act — to do his or her duty — simply because it is the right thing to do, with no thought for personal reward or punishment at any time or from any source.

The foundation of karma yoga can be summed up by the Golden Rule:

> *So in everything, do to others what you would have them do to you, for this sums up the Law and the Prophets*
> Matthew 7:12 (NIV)

The last clause of that quotation, "for this sums up the Law and the Prophets," can be read as "because it's the right thing to do."

Much of yoga is focused inward for the personal improvement and development of the body, mind, and spirit of the yogin. While karma yoga does indeed contribute to this process, it does so by directing the yogin to look outward and to act selflessly for the good of others, and to do so objectively without prejudice or pressure.

The outward gaze and subsequent actions are not to be limited to those of our own species, but are to extend to all of Creation. All things — from smallest to largest; those things we call "living" as well as those we call "non-living" — are united by the energetic frequencies of Creation that hold all things inseparably together.

Perform the tasks that fall within the sphere of your life; that is, do your job. Then do a little more. Look around you, observe your surroundings in the moment, and do the right thing with no thought of future consequences; then you will be a Karma Yogin.

Exercise

Besides the postures, a regular routine of exercise is also encouraged. You don't have to lift weights for hours on end, or run ten miles a day to build up strength and endurance; regular practice and mastery of the asanas will see to that. The exercise that best compliments the yogic postures is plain old walking. Walking was good enough for Gandhi, who walked several miles every day of his life. It is also the exercise most recommended by health care professionals, as well as yoga teachers. There is nothing like it for promoting good health, and there is no danger of injury or stress to the physical body.

For optimal physical health the yogin need look no further than the asanas, pranayama, and walking.

Materialism

> *¹⁹ Do not store up for yourselves treasures on earth, where moths and vermin destroy, and where thieves break in and steal. ²⁰ But store up for yourselves treasures in heaven, where moths and vermin do not destroy, and thieves do not break in and steal. ²¹ For where your treasure is, there your heart will be also.*
> Matthew 6:19-21 (NIV)

You've seen those storage facilities with row upon row of garage-like units that can be rented by the month. All you have to do is fill one up with your stuff and put a lock on it. It started here in the US in the 1960s, slowly at first, then took off in the 90s to become a multimillion–dollar industry. There are now nearly twice as many self-storage facilities in the US as there are Starbucks and McDonald's combined. In the rest of the world—particularly Great Britain and Western Europe—the trend to put things into storage rather than let go of them is growing. Just how much stuff do you really need anyway? If you have put something into storage and haven't thought of it in five years, do you really need it? If you don't need it, then why haven't you sold it or given it away? Do you own your stuff, or does your stuff own you? As a yogin, you should consider your possessions and potential acquisitions and ask, "Is this object necessary for—or will it get in the way of—my spiritual advancement?"

Once again, you are not expected to adopt the austere life of an ascetic; that would be not only contrary to the concept of moderation, but it would take all the fun out of life as well, and having fun is also a part of yoga. Be discriminant in your acquisitions, and don't become attached to them. Use them and enjoy them, but be ready to set them aside as your understanding grows and your needs change.

Study

How many times have you come home at the end of the day feeling drained of all your energy? You've spent all day solving problems, working out issues, and dealing with other people; all you want to do now is to relax and think of nothing.

Rather than turning on the television and letting the chaos of the nightly news, or the fake drama, forced humor and profanity of network programing wash over you, practice the niyama of swadhyaya (self-study) and pick up a good book instead. What better way to shed the stress of the day than to spend a half hour or so with the Bible, or the Gita, or the words of Yogananda, Thomas Merton, Krishnamurti, Thomas a'Kempis, Billy Graham, or other enlightened writer, regardless of their religious affiliation? Reflection on these types of writings will help to guide and ground you on your own spiritual path.

You could also study something entirely new and different, or pursue a life-long interest—something in the sciences, art, or history; make plans for next season's vegetable garden, or for landscaping to attract wildlife—the possibilities are endless.

There are people on this planet who have been looking for aliens to make contact with Earth. That will never happen as long as the human species remains stuck in the quagmire of what passes for entertainment on this planet. If you were an alien from a highly advanced civilization and you caught a glimpse of the Kardashians in action, or a half-hour of the nightly news, would you land on Earth? I think not. You would speed on by as fast as your little spaceship could take you and head for another star system altogether. With that in mind, you might consider your practice of swadhyaya to be your contribution toward interstellar relations.

Observe

By cultivating the ability to be an unbiased and careful observer, you can master all the other spiritual and mental principles of yoga; well-developed observational skills are especially important for the practice of karma yoga. You must learn to observe the events around you, not react to them. Don't allow yourself to get attached to anything in the home, at work, or in the wider world. Everything on this planet is, to a certain extent, an illusion that will pass away. Nothing is worth the time and energy it takes to worry about it. Distance yourself from the illusion. Distance yourself from those around you who are short-tempered, vain, evil, self-centered, and worldly.

The writings of spiritual leaders from the Saints, Apostles, and Billy Graham, to Yogananda and Krishnamurti instruct you to separate yourselves from negative influences, including people. Simply observe and walk away. Be like Kwai Chang Caine (Grasshopper); be an observer.

Observe, but don't let things get to you; don't build roadblocks in your yogic path. You will find that the more practiced you become with the postures, the breathing, and the meditation and prayer—the longer you are on the path of yoga—the easier it will be to take on the role of the observer. When that occurs, you will be able to practice the principles of karma yoga to the fullest extent. By becoming detached, you will be able to assess each situation logically and without bias; you will know when to step in and what help to offer. Others will be drawn to you for guidance and direction, which you will now be able to give freely and lovingly.

But the yogi who has disciplined the mind and has control of the senses can move about amidst sense objects, free of attraction and aversion, settling more deeply in tranquility.
Bhagavad Gita 2:64; *The Living Gita, A commentary for modern readers*, by Sri Swami Satchidananda

Note: There are many translations and interpretations of the Bhagavad Gita; the one cited for this quotation is my personal favorite, and is highly recommended as a straight-forward and accurate translation with notes and commentary that do not overburden the text.

Conclusion

You are now ready to walk the yogic path of life. I predict that after a few short months you will never go back to your old way of life. Just remember two important things:

First, you must not give up after only a few weeks or a few yoga sessions. Pour yourself into the lifestyle, and think of yourself as a True Yogic Warrior who walks this earth as an objective observer. Take the yamas and niyamas seriously and live the life of a jivanmukta—one who is liberated while still in the body.

Second, enjoy life and have fun along your way. Laugh and smile more, whether it seems natural at first or not. As a yogin there is nothing to frown about and much to be joyful for.

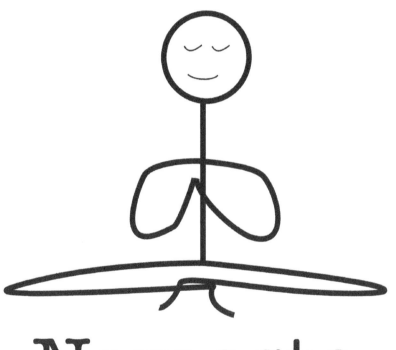

Namaste

Made in the USA
Coppell, TX
17 February 2022

73698625R00090